Green Smoothie

Diet, Detox and Recipes

Ellen Vincent

First Printing, 2012

ISBN-13: 978-1475179736

ISBN-10: 1475179731

Printed in the United States of America

Dedication

To almighty God and my husband Tim

Green Smoothie

Diet, Detox and Recipes

Table of Contents

Introduction

Most of us struggle with our health, to a certain extent, even if we say that we are generally healthy. I used to keep getting colds for example and sometimes my skin was really dry and sore on the back of my hands. I have also struggled with my weight. As with most people this has become more of a problem as I have gotten older. There were also some days that I just didn't seem to have the energy to do anything. Some weeks have been a problem in particular and those are when I am on holiday and away from the usual stresses of work. It is terrible being tired when you are on holiday because it stops you doing all of the things that make life pleasurable. Who wouldn't rather be more awake, full of life and free from those niggling little conditions? Well, this book is all about getting your body working the best that it can. Little did I know a few years ago that the first step towards this new healthy paradigm was to drink just one green smoothie a day.

The normal diet that people eat these days shows little resemblance to the food that our ancestors would have eaten in the early stages of human existence. We are used to a world of plenty where as our ancestors had to make do with what they could find. Meat was something that would have been very irregular so people would have relied upon the various leaves and fruits that they could find. Certainly they would have consumed far more vegetation than we currently have in our modern diets. There can be great benefits gained from increasing the amount of green leaves and fruits in our diets. Vegetables add valuable roughage to our diet which enables the digestive system to work the way nature intended. This in itself will help us feel better as well as helping to avoid such modern diseases as bowl cancer. The green leaves that we consume also provide valuable nutrients in the form of minerals and vitamins. As well as this, leaves are low in fats. This is good because excess fats from meats and dairy produce are the curse of the modern Western diet. This is the reason that so many people in the West struggle with maintaining a healthy weight.

One of the main problems with increasing your intake of leafy greens is that they appear to be so dull compared to all of the other high fat foods that surround us from day to day. Who wouldn't be tempted to have a juicy steak or a cheese pie rather than a stick of celery and a leaf from a cabbage? Green smoothies solve this problem by combining the natural green aspect of leaves with the natural flavours and sweetness of fruits. Fruits such as bananas or mangoes can add much needed flavour to your green smoothie. Once the fruit is all mixed up with the greens in the smoothie you will just have an overall flavour to deal with, and so long as this is pleasant you haven't got to think about the dull taste of such things as spinach or broccoli.

The other thing about eating a whole lot of green leaves and other raw vegetation is that you will have to chew them a lot in order to get the nutrients out of them. Animals that eat only leaves have to spend a whole lot of their time just chewing and re-chewing their food, before they swallow it, so that they can get all of the good stuff out of it. With a green smoothie all of this chewing has already been done for you by the blender that you use. The pieces of the leaves and vegetables are shredded into very small bits and this helps to release all of the goodness out of them. You can then simply swallow the smoothie, like you would a fruit juice, and then get on with your life.

The nutrients in leaves and other vegetation are trapped within plant cells that have resilient cell walls around them for protection and structure. The idea of chewing, and the same for the blender, is that the soluble nutrients within the cells are released so that they can be digested and then absorbed from the gut to be transported around the body in the blood stream. The blade action of the blender will release the contents from many cells increasing the amount of nutrients that can be utilized by the body. Normally if you fail to chew raw vegetables and swallow large chunks of them the cells do not release their contents and the valuable nutrients just pass through the whole of the digestive system and are egested from the body. The reason for this is that our digestive system doesn't have the necessary digestive enzymes to deal with the cellulose in the cell walls. As a result they will remain intact and keep their contents from being used as nutrients.

Herbivores which utilise vegetation as the whole of their diet use bacteria to produce enzymes to break down the cellulose walls. In actual fact, these cellulose walls are very energy rich and it is just that we, as humans, haven't got any way of dealing them. In the dim and dark distant past this wasn't necessarily true because we still have the organ that used to do this particular work. What I am talking about is the appendix. This was the part that dealt with cell walls, but in modern humans it just doesn't work. This doesn't mean to say that your appendix will magically start doing this job if you eat lots of vegetation. This really can't happen now and was probably only functioning in some of our distant lines of evolution. The fact that we can't digest cellulose like a rabbit is in actual fact a good thing because it means that all the cell walls that can't be digested add bulk to our food. This is what we call fibre or roughage.

Green smoothies also contain a lot of vitamins which means that you don't need spend extra money on supplements in the form of tablets or capsules. Natural vitamins are always a better choice than the refined ones in tablets which come packaged with other undesirables such as refined sugar and artificial colours. Getting your vitamins from a pure natural source has always got to be the right choice.

Green leaves also contain a wealth of antioxidants and these too are very valuable for the body. They are used to deal with pollutants and other undesirable chemicals which can cause the cells of the body to age prematurely.

As well as all of these fantastic natural ingredients green smoothies should also be considered good for what they leave out. Unlike a lot of shop bought drinks, you make your green smoothies from fruit and vegetables that have come direct from the field and this means that they won't contain such things as artificial sweeteners, preservatives or flavour enhancers. All of these things can have a negative affect on our lives and should be avoided if possible. Green smoothies that you make at home are the perfect way to avoid these food additives and the problems that they bring.

One barrier to drinking these kinds of smoothies is the colour. They are green, and often bright green. To a lot of people drinks of this colour and consistency just don't seem to be right. Maybe it reminds them of green slime ore something like that? You have to try and get beyond this initial vision of the green smoothie and think about the actual flavour. So long as you have mixed the green leaves with fruit then you will have a smoothie that is full of flavour as well as goodness. The colour will often defy the fact that they are usually made up of more fruit than greens. The typical ratio is somewhere in the region of 40 percent greens and 60 percent fruit. The dominant flavour is therefore more on the fruit side. I am sure that after you have had a couple of green smoothies you won't even think about the colour and consistency again. You can also change the colour to a more appealing red by adding beetroot or red cabbage, if you think that this would make a difference to you.

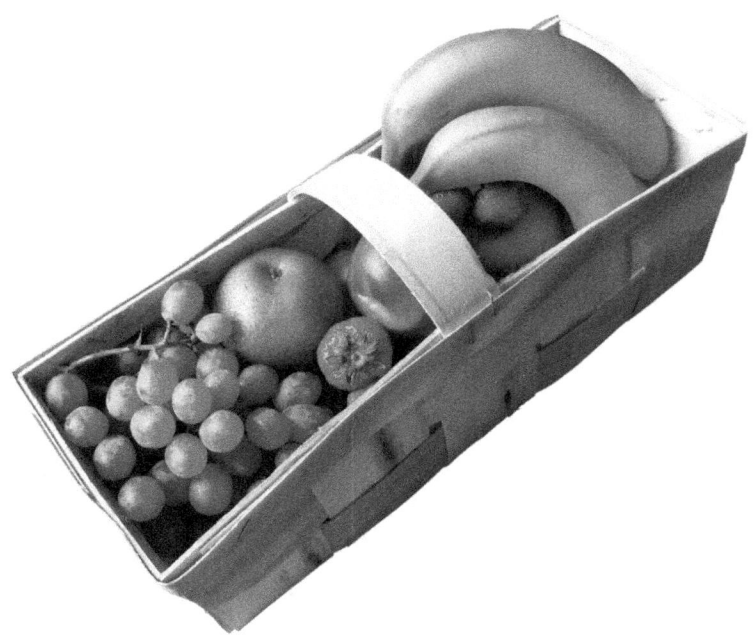

Typical fruits added to green smoothies include strawberries, bananas, raspberries and blueberries. However, you can add all kinds of fruit depending on your desire and what is available locally. The fact that green smoothies contain mainly such fruits is the reason why they taste so good. The addition of green vegetables then gives the extra healthy edge that will make the difference to your life. Green smoothies contain far more nutrition when you compare them to a smoothie made entirely from fruit alone.

The health benefits of green smoothies

Health bodies and the government have really been pushing the idea that people should consume at least 5 portions of fruit and vegetables a day. This idea is sound, but it is often difficult to get around to eating these amounts. After 1 portion of fruit, the next one is ok, but after that people tend to forget about it. As for vegetables they tend to be left on the side of the plate especially if we aren't feeling up to eating very much. Green smoothies are an ideal way of getting to your 5 a day and more. They taste so good that you don't realize how much fruit and greens that you are actually eating. Added to this is the fact that the greens are uncooked and as a result have much more value in terms of vitamin and antioxidant content.

A green smoothie is a tasty food item to drink but that isn't the end of it. Once you start having green smoothies as a part of your normal diet you will find that there are many different benefits that you will experience. Even after a short amount of time you will find that you will seem to have increased levels of energy and a general feeling of well being.

In the longer term green smoothies can be used to help lose weight and prevent the onset of many health conditions including the chronic ones that often blight people's lives. As well as this, people have also found that, with a green smoothie diet, it doesn't take as long to recover from illnesses and injuries and that they have more stamina and energy when doing sporting activities. The more that green smoothies become a part of your life the greater that you will notice that your general health improves.

Artificial sweeteners have still not been cleared as far as their abilities to cause cancers and as a result avoiding them is a good thing. Some artificial sweeteners have also been linked to a greater instance of heart disease. Even if the sweetener is a simple sugar it will have been refined from the natural versions into syrup. These sugars don't come with their related cells and as a result they can hit the blood stream very quickly and cause vast increases in blood sugar levels. This in turn can lead to a greater risk of becoming diabetic. These huge increases in sugar lead to people becoming resistant to their own insulin and eventually can cause type 2 diabetes. However, when the sugars are trapped within cells they are released more slowly and this means that there are fewer peaks in blood sugar levels once they are absorbed from the gut.

The extra fibre in green smoothies has quite a number of health benefits. It can make us feel full as well as giving the circular muscles in our gut something to contract against to move the food through our digestive system. This fact means that conditions like constipation and colon cancer are far less likely to happen. Constipation can cause a lot of pain in people that suffer from it and the fact that the food lingers in the large intestine means that it will start to break down due to the actions of bacteria in the gut. These bacteria can release toxins and other chemicals which can induce cancer. It is therefore very important to make sure that the food travels through the digestive system at an even rate and is egested on a regular basis. The extra fibre included in these smoothies is one important reason that they are better for you than just drinking the juices. Juicing is still popular, and rightfully so, because freshly juiced fruits and vegetables do contain valuable vitamins and minerals. However, why consume just juice when you can have a green smoothie and include all of that useful fibre as well?

Fibre in the diet can also help in the maintaining of blood sugar levels. This is important for people with pre-diabetes and those who have to try and control diabetes with dietary restrictions. The fibre tends to hang onto sugars that have been digested in the gut. This means that they are only slowly released to be absorbed into the blood through the gut wall. This then helps to reduce peaks in blood sugar levels. This could mean the difference between taking tablets or not taking tablets to control a person's diabetes. This is important because the tablets involved in diabetes treatment often have side effects that can lead to a poorer experience of life.

Green smoothies can also help in controlling cholesterol levels in the blood as well. To start off with, green smoothies contain low amounts of cholesterol and fatty materials compared to meat and dairy products. The human body itself is able to manufacture its own cholesterol from basic food building blocks, so there is very little need to include extra cholesterol in a normal diet. Meat and dairy based foods contain far too many cholesterol elements and as a result we are often advised by health experts to cut down on the amounts that we consume.

Not all cholesterol is the same. There are in fact two different types that are important for humans. They are used in such processes as the manufacture of cell membranes, cell reproduction and dealing with stress. Our bodies need both kinds of cholesterol but in the right proportions. So long as we maintain these proportions we will be healthy. Low density lipoproteins or LDL cholesterol has been given the dubious characterization as being the bad cholesterol whereas High density lipoproteins or HDL cholesterol is said to be the good cholesterol. The liver tries to maintain a ratio of 4 parts LDL cholesterol to 10 parts HDL cholesterol. At this point both are in balance and the body functions well. Problems arise if the ratio drops to 3 parts LDL to 10 parts HDL. Once this happens the HDL bad cholesterol starts to deposit fatty materials on the inner walls of arteries. These can build up to form plaques which can restrict the flow of blood through these blood vessels. This condition is known as arteriosclerosis. If the plaques are formed in the thin coronary artery, which supplies the heart with nutrients, then a heart attack can occur. This is then called coronary heart disease. These plaques can also cause blood clots to form which then can cause strokes if they lodge in the brain. It is therefore important to maintain the correct balance of good to bad cholesterol. The good LDL cholesterol can help prevent the fatty plaques forming in arteries where as the bad HDL cholesterol speeds up the plaque build up.

Green smoothies work in 2 ways to help maintain the ratio of good to bad cholesterol in the blood. Firstly they contain very little cholesterol and therefore the liver can do its job and create the correct ratio of the cholesterols. Secondly the roughage, in the form of all of the plant cells walls made of cellulose, tends to absorb and hang onto fatty materials in the diet. This then makes them less likely to be absorbed from the gut and enter the blood stream. This means that, even if you only have one green smoothie a day and then have normal meals the rest of the day, the extra roughage will help prevent the blood taking up excess fats from the digested food.

Green smoothies are a completely natural food supplied to your body the way nature intended. Cooking is really an artificial way of preparing food that was developed by man. No other animals on the planet actually prepare their food in this way. The further we go away from what nature intended the more problems that we have. For example, people in Africa who have more natural food have less tooth decay and basically stronger teeth. Here in the West our teeth are weak and prone to decay and gum disease. People who come to the West from Africa start to suffer these tooth and gum disease once they start on the typical Western Diet of cooked soft food.

By keeping green smoothies as a part of your diet you will see that your body will react in a lot of positive ways. Many people have reported that they have more energy to do the things that they want to; less aches and pains from their body; better sleeping and less insomnia; increased sexual desire; more active thinking and alertness; fewer illnesses and illnesses that last a shorter amount of time; clearer skin including reduced acne and eczema; reduced cravings for caffeine containing drinks and more regular bowel movements. This all adds up to a better mind and a better body.

The green colour in green plants is produced by the chlorophyll molecule which is very similar in structure to the haemoglobin in our blood cells. This means that chlorophyll contains the basic building blocks to make new blood cells. As a result all you need to add is the element iron to the diet and you then have a perfect food to help you with tiredness and anaemia. Green smoothies can therefore help to increase the number of red blood cells in circulation.

The chlorophyll molecule has magnesium at the centre of its structure and therefore this mineral element is supplied in high levels when green smoothies are consumed. Magnesium is an important mineral because it can help to relieve cravings that you might get for such things as fatty snacks including cakes, biscuits and chocolate. .

19

The calcium provided by such greens as kale and dandelion is very important for the maintenance of bones and teeth. By selecting your greens carefully you can increase the content of particular minerals and hence tailor your smoothies to your needs.

How to make a green smoothie

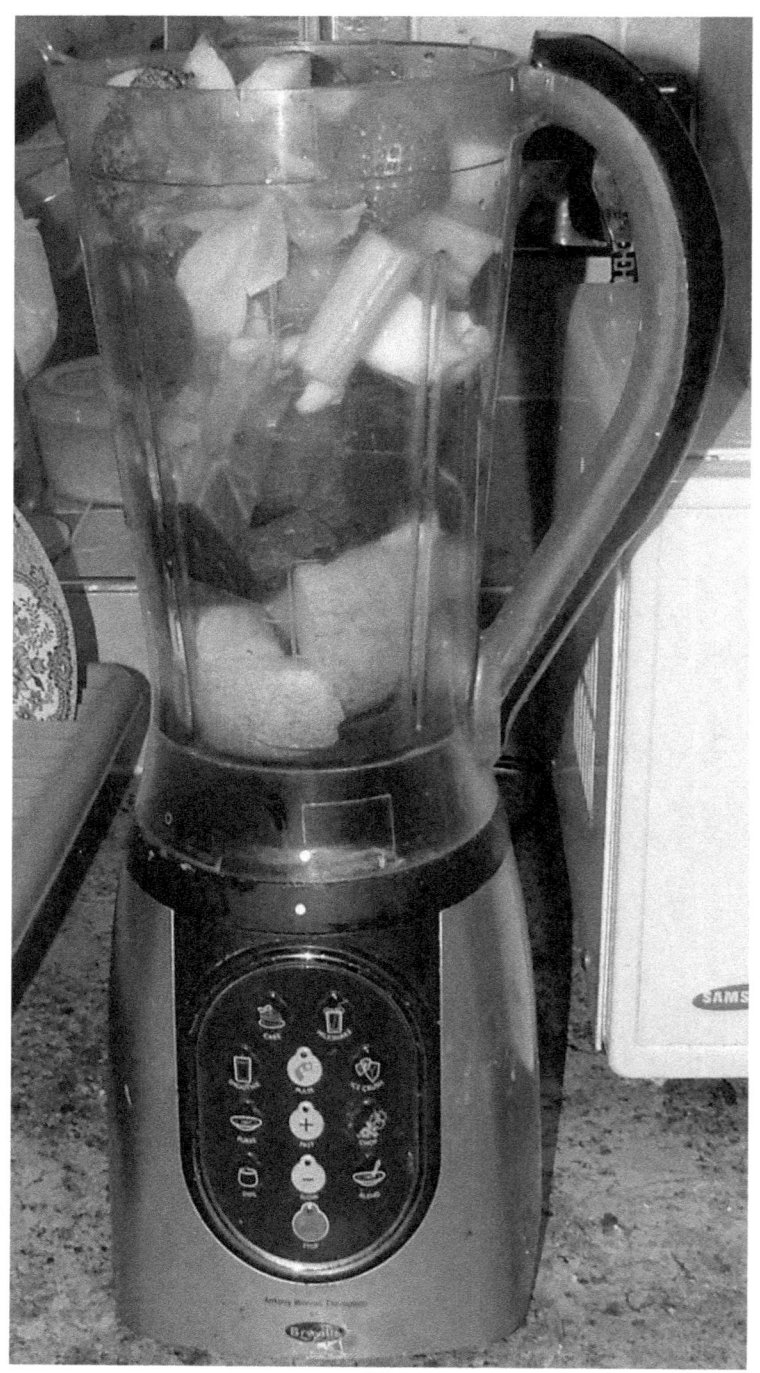

The essential part of your armoury is a high speed blender designed to make smoothies. I have one that can be programmed for a number of tasks including a smoothie setting. This does the job really well. It is simply a case of pressing the smoothie button on the blender. Nothing could be simpler. Beware of really cheap blenders because they may not have the speed to chop all the vegetables up and you will end up with lots of large chunks instead of a really smooth consistency.

Select the fruits and greens that you want to use in your smoothie. Try to make it that there is about 60% fruit and 40% greens. The best tasting smoothies tend to use only a few different fruits so that the flavours really come out. Try different combinations but you could start with fruits such as banana, strawberries and mangoes which have very definite flavours.

Wash the fruit and chop it into chunks. Don't just throw in the whole fruit, especially if it is large because this may prevent the rest of the fruit reaching the blades. Put the fruit into the blender and then add water until the fruit is covered. The type of water is really up to you. Tap water has added chlorine so I often use bottled water instead. I also like to use coconut water. This is the water from inside a fresh coconut. These days you can often get fresh coconuts from the local market or specialist African shops in towns. Some people use fresh spring water but this according to its availability. If you are using spring water make sure that it is fit for human consumption and hasn't got farm run off in it which may include pesticides, fertilizers and even animal waste. You can also try using fruit juices instead of water for a richer tasting smoothie. Make sure that the juices you use are 100% fruit juice. Avoid cartons which say 'nectar' or 'drink' as these often have added refined sugar.

Take a selection of fresh green leafy vegetables. You could include such vegetables as kale, spinach, parsley, bok choy, lettuce, cabbage, broccoli and even the green parts from the dandelion plant. Romaine lettuce is a good choice because it contains a good array of nutrients. Romaine lettuce is known as Cos lettuce in other parts of the world. Fill the rest of the space in the blender with the greens and then blend until the mixture is nice and smooth. Drink the smoothie straight away and start to reap the benefits of your new lifestyle.

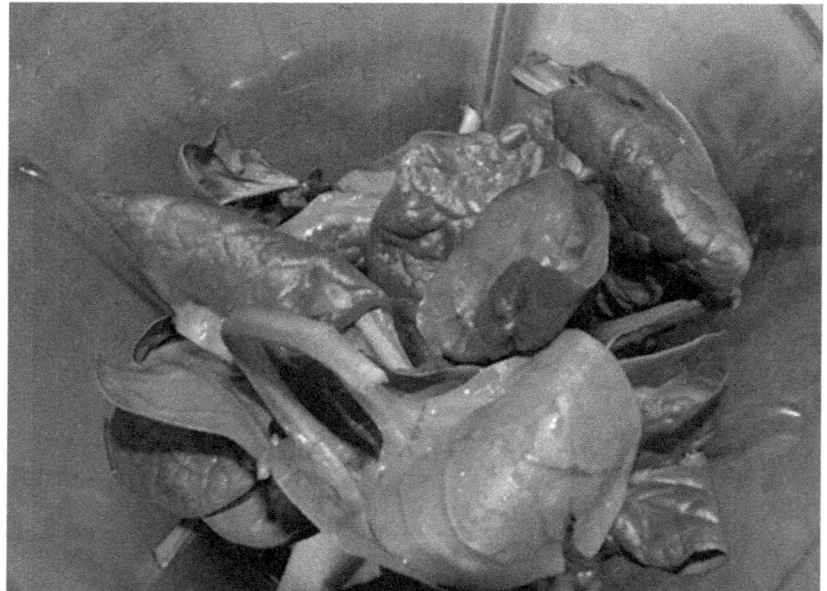

Young Spinach leaves in the blender

To start off with, keep your smoothies quite simple using only fruits, fresh leafy green vegetables and water. You should find that these will be easier to digest than more complicated smoothie mixtures involving seeds and nuts. You could also try and use organic produce as this should be free from pesticide and inorganic fertilizer residues. If you are using ordinary fruit and vegetables then make sure that they are thoroughly washed before using them.

Peeling any root vegetables can also reduce any pesticides that may have become adsorbed onto the surface.

In terms of nutrients, kale is thought to contain the most concentrated amounts. In terms of fruits, berries are a very good choice because they have lots of healthy anti oxidants and the sugars that they contain have a low direct affect on blood sugar levels.

It is best to consume your smoothie straight away after you have made it. The reason for this is that some vitamins start to degenerate as soon as they are exposed to oxygen in the air. Vitamin C in particular is prone to degeneration after blending. Adding some lemon juice can help with this as the acid conditions provided by the lemon juice tend to stabilize the vitamin C preventing its degeneration.

Try to rotate the vegetables that you use in your smoothies each day. The reason for this is that vegetables contain alkaloids. These substances are in small quantities and are part of the plants natural defence mechanism against animals that might eat them. You can consider them as being 'mustard like' and they are the reason that some vegetables have a slight mustard flavour. These shouldn't do any harm to the human body but as different plants contain different alkaloids rotation prevents the build up of any particular one.

If you have a blender with a narrow bottom you may find that the blades pin round but they don't reach the food above. You can try putting the water in first because this will help the blades to do their job and draw in the chunks of food from above. You can also try using the blender pulse feature to try and encourage the solid lumps of food to move back towards the blades as they spin around. Blenders with a pre-programmed smoothie button will often do this as a matter of course to ensure that the food is blended evenly.

When you first start eating green smoothies you may find that the taste of the added green leaves a bit much and as a result it is a good idea to add some extra berries to your recipe. These will give added taste and natural sweetness to your smoothie which will make it more appealing. To make green smoothies go down a bit easier in the early days of using them you can add some ice cubes. This will tend to dull the more extreme flavours and allow you to drink them more easily.

Here are 2 smoothie recipes that I have made recently and show the great variations that you can make in producing interesting green drinks

Cabbage cocktail

Savoy Cabbage leaves
½ apple
Juice of half lemon
1 carrot
1 kiwi
3 radish
6 strawberries
3 celery ribs
Dried apricots
1 banana

Rosy red relish

Spinach
1 beetroot
1 carrot
1 apple
5 strawberries
Juice of 1 Lemon with some water

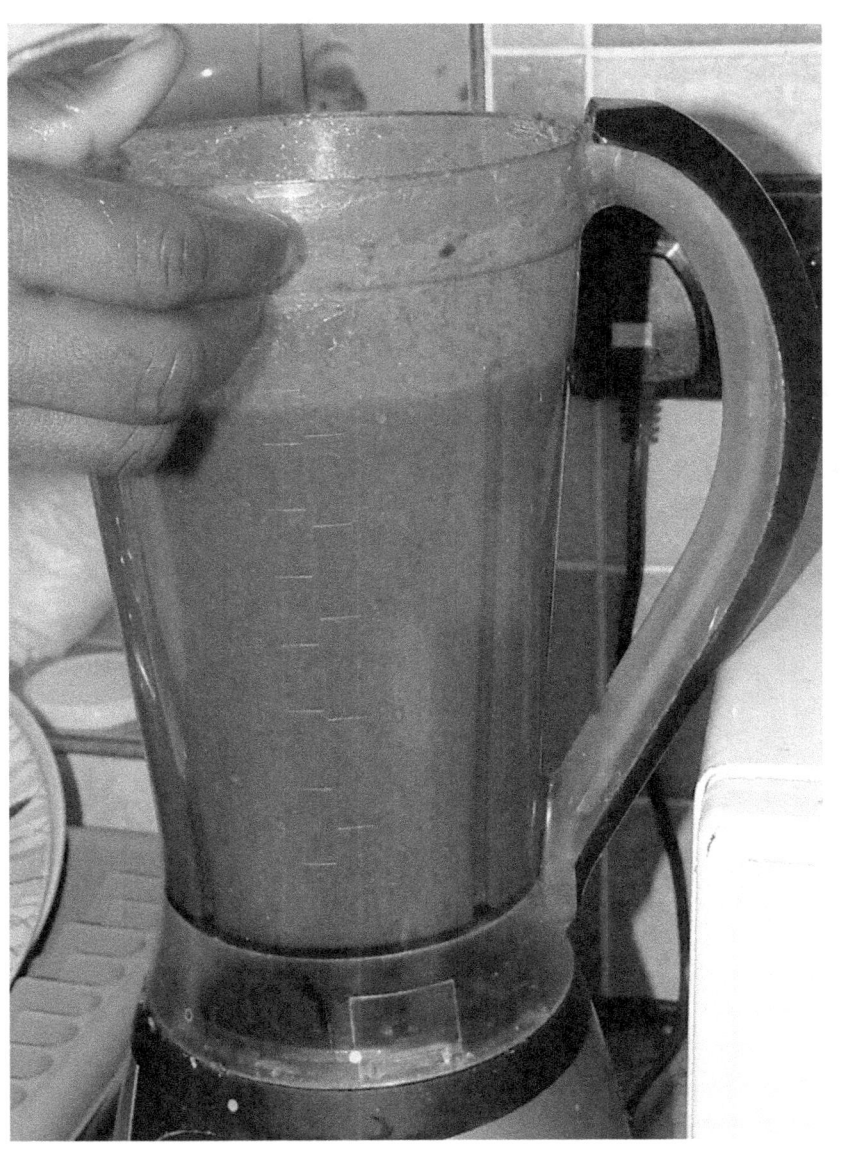

Green smoothie nutrition facts

When you look at the nutrients in green smoothies you begin to see why they are such a valuable part of a person's diet. A lot of the benefits gained from green smoothies come about due to the large amounts of fibre and antioxidants that the vegetable leaves contain. In addition to this, green smoothies also contain a lot of health giving vitamins, minerals and other factors. Examples of these are:

Calcium
Potassium
Iron
Magnesium
Manganese
Zinc
Copper
Vitamin C
Vitamin K
Vitamin A
Vitamin E
Vitamin B2
Vitamin B3
Vitamin B5
Vitamin B6
Vitamin B6
Folate
Tryptophan
Omega 3 fatty acids

These elements provided by green smoothies are all important for the correct running of the body. Vitamin deficiencies, for example, can have dire consequences for an individual. In the past individuals suffered the condition scurvy due to the lack of fresh fruit and vegetables in their diet. The body just literally drops to pieces with this condition. Sailors on old fashioned sailing boats used to suffer this disease when they were at sea for many months. The introduction of fruit to their diet soon improved the situation. Vitamin deficiencies aren't a thing of the past. There are great worries at the moment that children aren't getting enough vitamin D in their diet and that the condition known as rickets has returned to affect the growth of bones in young people. As you can see vitamins are really important and getting them from a natural source is better than any tablets that you might take.

Even though the nutrients loaded into green smoothies are central to how they work, we should also consider those things that aren't in them. In particular, there are many unhealthy items that are left out. These things include the saturated, trans-saturated fats and cholesterol which increase the risk of coronary heart disease and strokes; refined sugars such as fructose syrup which can elevate blood sugar levels and lead to type 2 diabetes; artificial colours and flavours which can cause hyperactivity in children and possibly cancers; mono sodium glutamate flavour enhancers which can cause various problems with the nervous system and hormones from animals which can have dramatic effects on the body including weight gain and sexual problems. The list could continue on with many other problem substances. It has also been established that cooking foods can also change some food ingredients into cancer producing substances.

Green smoothies are therefore so much healthier than the foods that we are used to consuming on a daily basis. This will mean a genuine health boost if you continue having green smoothies on a daily basis.

With vegetarian diets there is always a concern about the levels of protein that is provided. The best way of supplying this is to have a varied diet of different protein sources. You can select those vegetables that are higher in protein such as broccoli and spinach. You can also add other plant material which is high in protein such as nuts. These too will easily chop up and add to your green smoothie. In addition to this the cell contents released by blending green vegetables contain amino acids and proteins in the form of live enzymes.

Although it is possible to survive on just a green smoothie diet this is not necessarily recommended by most advocates of green smoothies. It is probably better to have a mixed diet where you have smoothies to start off the day and then have some regular meals later on. The green smoothies will still do their job of providing the natural ingredients with extra vitamins, minerals and antioxidants but the other parts of your diet will provide the extra protein that you may feel that you need. You could then gradually increase the amount of green smoothies that you consume until you feel happy with the results that you are getting. You will also find that without the cravings for snacks and a feeling of being full you will be less likely to want to eat huge amounts at other meal times.

Green leaves are also a source of omega 3 unsaturated fats. These are known to be good for us and usually we struggle to have the right amounts of these essential fats. The usual route is to take supplements or eat oily fish. Green leaves and seeds such as those of the flax plant are equally good sources of these omega 3 fats. Some people consider flax to be a bit difficult to eat but in a smoothie you wouldn't notice it. Fatty alternatives to flax seeds include chia seeds or avocado. Chia seeds have a good ratio of omega 3 to omega 6 essential fatty acids and are therefore a good choice.

Greens are also relatively low in usable carbohydrate. This is because the carbohydrate that makes up the structure of these leaves is not really available to us. The fruit, however, that you add to the green smoothie contains a lot of usable carbohydrate and therefore provides the energy that your body needs to do its daily activities. All of the sugar in fruits is trapped within cells and it takes time for it to get released and digested. This means that the sugars get slowly released unlike foods that have added sugar syrup. As a result it doesn't have a huge sudden impact on your blood sugar levels. Slow release sugars like these are far better for us and therefore don't result in the insulin tolerance that leads to type 2 diabetes.

Selecting the greens

You should choose greens which are dark in colour because these generally have the most protein in them. You can choose from those greens that are easy to obtain from the supermarket or those that grow as edible weeds in your garden or round about in your neighbourhood. You should take care to only pick the weeds that are edible. Here are some of the common ones:

Dandelion

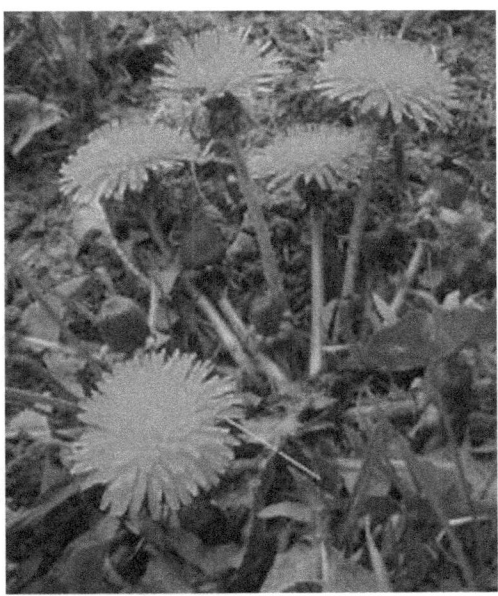

This is one of the greens that is a common weed. We see these plants all about us in the spring and summer growing in all kinds of areas. I have them growing in my lawn for example and I can also find them in the park. They are everywhere and they are free. You can also buy them from health stores as well. Dandelion leaves have lots of vitamins including A and K. They also have a lot of calcium and iron mineral content. In fact there are more of these nutrients in dandelion leaves than in spinach or broccoli.

Dandelion greens can help digestion to take place and also act as part of a system cleanse or detox. They can help with constipation because they also act as a natural laxative. This together with increased urine production helps in the removal of toxins from the body. They are also supposed to help in the fight against viruses as well as healing for eczema and acne.

When foraging for dandelion greens make sure that the area hasn't been treated with herbicides and pesticides. Roadsides will also be problem due to pollutants from the vehicles that use them.

Romaine or Cos lettuce

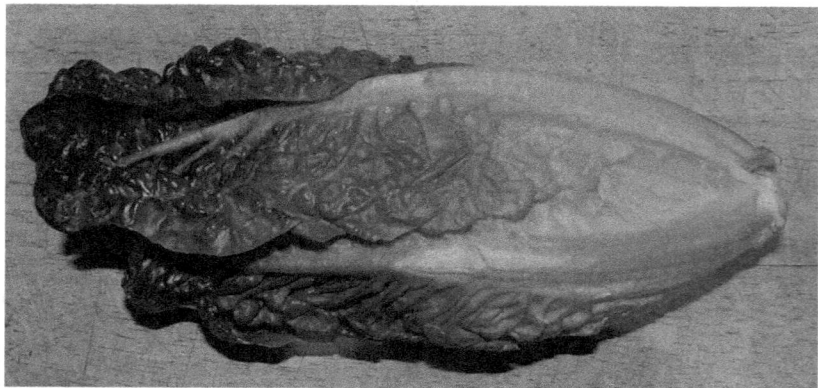

Cos Lettuce

This type of lettuce is very good for adding to smoothies. They are stuffed full of nutrients and have a high water content. The extra fibre in this lettuce is good for maintaining the movement of food through the gut and trapping fatty materials that would end up in the blood stream and affect heart health. The vitamins C, K and A are found in high levels. They are also a good source of folic acid and the minerals manganese and chromium.

Due to the fact that lettuce readily absorbs pesticides and other agricultural chemicals it is best to either buy organic versions or grow your own. Make sure you wash your lettuce well before using it in the smoothie.

Spinach

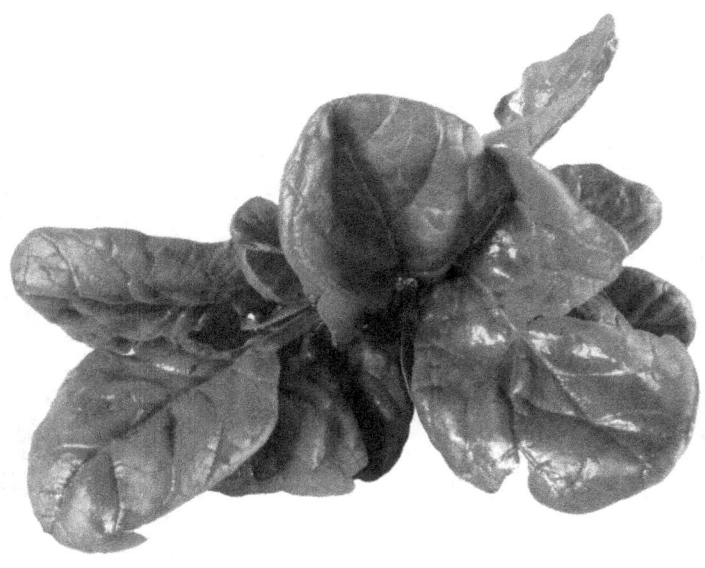

Spinach

Spinach is packed full of useful nutrients including lots of vitamins K, C, E and A. It is also full of calcium and magnesium minerals which when combined with the vitamin K is very good for the skeletal system. The mineral iron is also found in large amounts in spinach and this is good for making red blood cells and curing anaemia. It is packed full of flavenoids which help to protect the body against cancer. It is also believed to help with heart disease and Alzheimer's conditions.

Riboflavin in spinach can help with head aches and migraine. The vitamin E can help with skin conditions as well as giving clearer thinking. The carotenoid lutein is also present in spinach and this is good for the eyes and reinforces the retina against the condition known as macular degeneration.

Chard

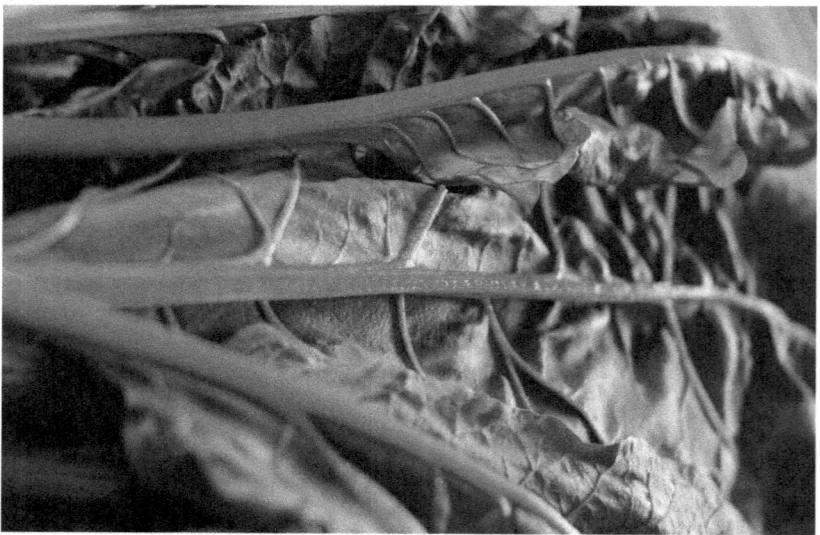

Swiss chard

Chard belongs to the group of vegetables known as beets. This includes beetroot which is obviously a root crop.

Chard on the other hand is grown for the nutritious leaves that are produced rather than the roots. The leaves are high in fibre and contains lots of the vitamins, A, C, E, B, E and K as well the minerals potassium, iron, magnesium, calcium, phosphorus and manganese. They are also high in protein content which is very desirable.

It is believed that Chard can help to prevent cancers. They are good at cleansing the gut as well as supporting the immune and skeletal systems. Like spinach there is also lutein present for eye health. Chard leaves are slightly bitter in taste but a lot less bitter than other beet family leaves such as beetroot.

Broccoli

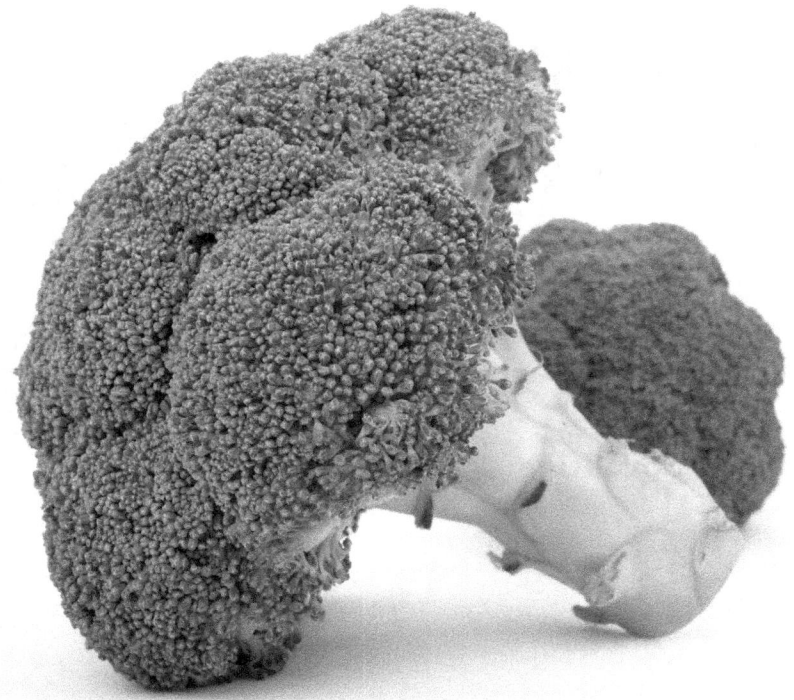

Broccoli

37

Broccoli has fantastic detoxifying properties. It helps to boost enzymes in the liver that then help to remove toxic substances from the body. It is rich in the vitamins K, C and A which all help to promote the immune system and deal with free radicals especially in the skin. This helps prevent cancers and aging of the cells. Calcium levels are also high in Broccoli and this can help in the maintenance of bones and teeth. Antioxidants and carotenoids in broccoli can help to prevent cancers. It also contains lutein which helps with eye health. You can also use purple sprouting which is a variety of broccoli with the same nutrient content. It is much more like the original broccoli plant and has purple florets and longer stems both of which are edible.

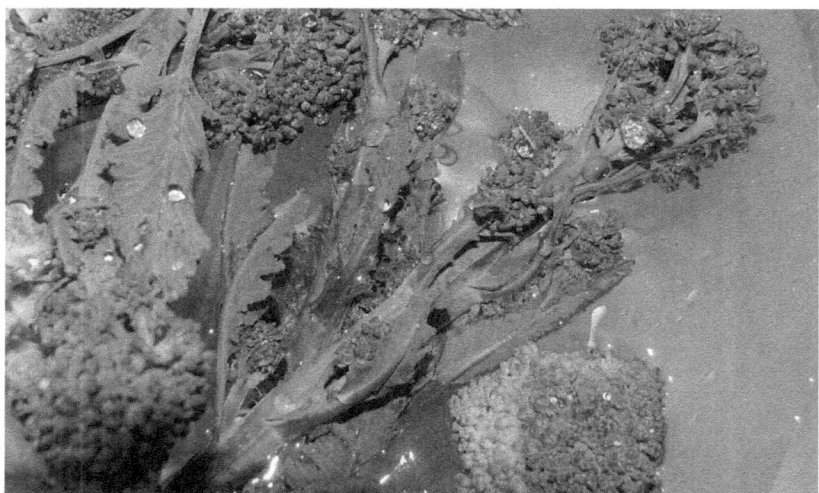

Purple Sprouting

Cabbage

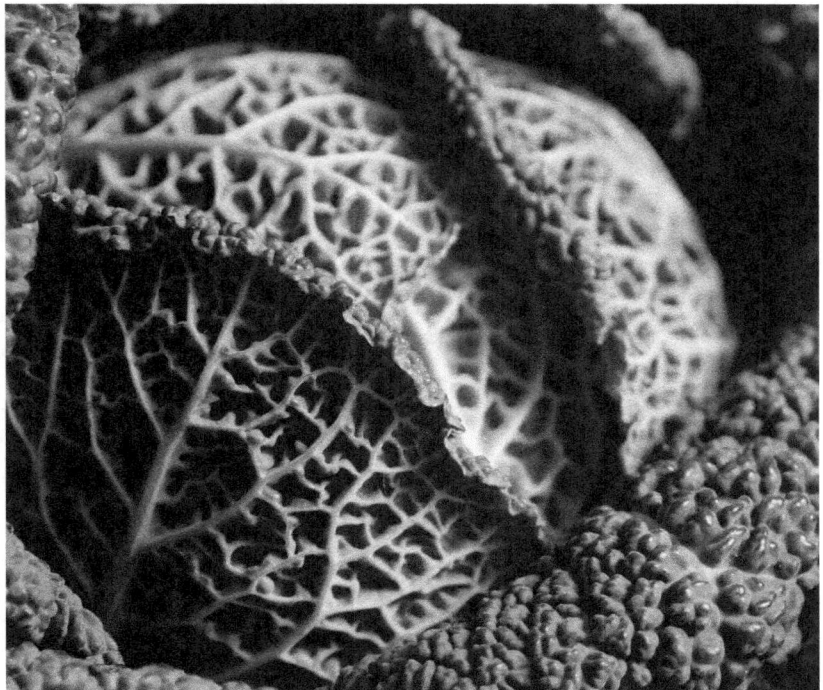

Savoy cabbage

Cabbage can help with detoxification routines. It can also help with preventing cancers. Cabbage has a lot of vitamin C and fibre and is therefore good at boosting the immune system as well as helping with constipation. It has properties which help it to deal with inflammation and as a result is considered to be helpful with arthritic conditions.

There are a number of different cabbage family greens that you can use including savoy, spring, bok choy and red cabbage. Red cabbage is also thought to help with preventing Alzheimer's and other kinds of dementia.

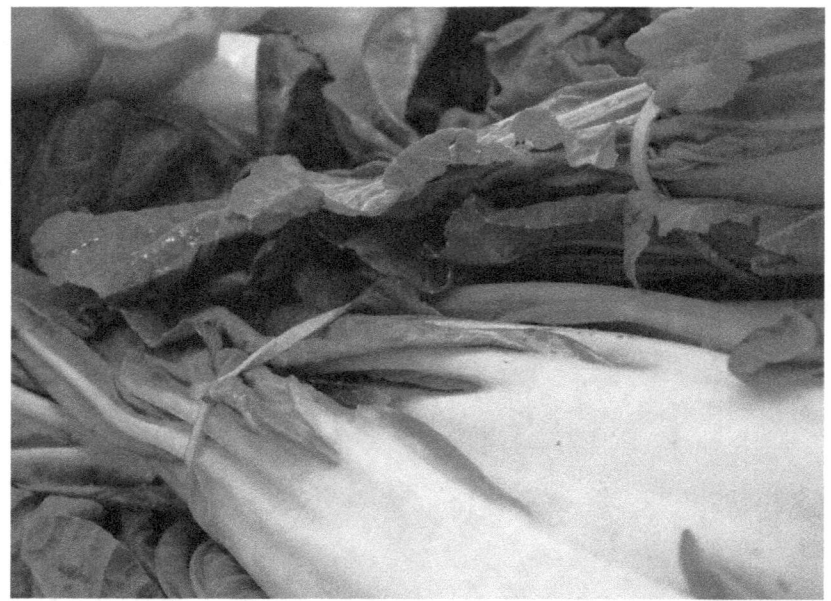

Bok Choy

Kale

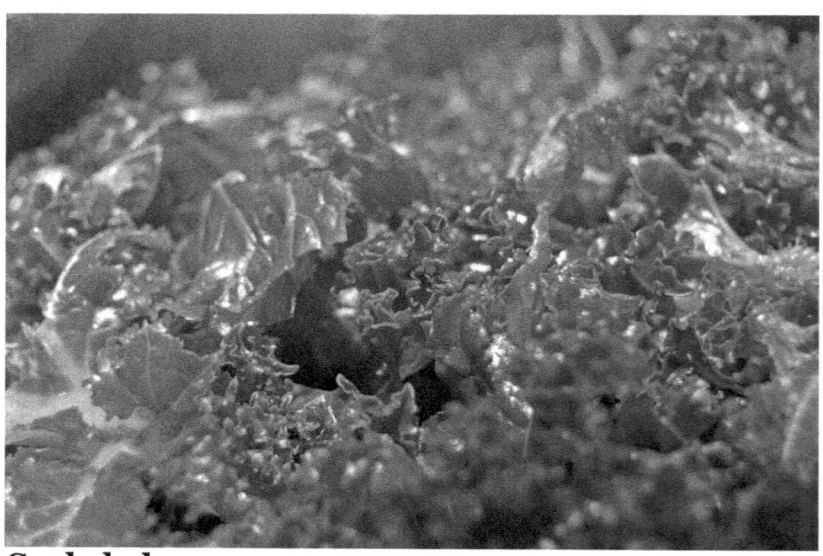

Curly kale

Kale is dark green leafed vegetable which is increasing in popularity around the world. In some areas however, it is still difficult to buy so you may have to look around a lot to find suitable sources. It has a fantastic richness of nutrients combined with a great flavour.

Raw Kale has been linked to a number of health benefits such as protecting against cancer and decreasing bad cholesterol levels. There are a number of different varieties of kale that you can find including curly and ornamental. Most importantly for green smoothie lovers is the fact that it is a good vegetable source of protein.

Kale contains a lot of fibre, calcium, magnesium, iron and phosphorus as well as the vitamins A, C, B6 and K. It also contains many antioxidants including carotenoids and flavenoids which help with protection against cancer. Kale also contains zeaxanthin and lutein which are good for the health of the eyes.

Parsley

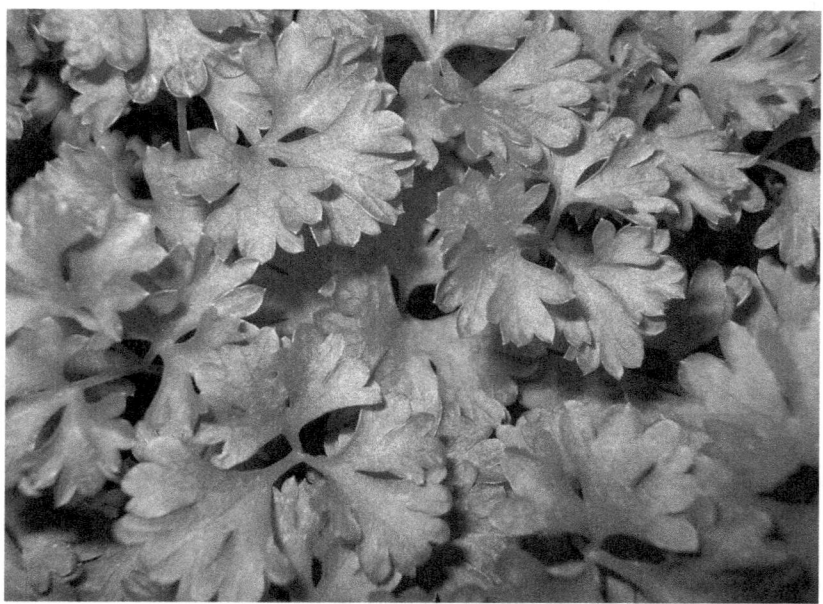

Parsley

Parsley is very rich in antioxidants, minerals, vitamins and fibre. It has no cholesterol in its make up. It also contains eugenol essential oil which can act as a local anaesthetic and antiseptic agent and has been used in dentistry. This oil has also been noted for decreasing blood sugar levels.

It has been described as the best plant source for flavenoid type antioxidants which are very good at dealing with free radicals that cause aging of body cells and cancer. It is also rich in the minerals potassium, iron, manganese and calcium as well as the vitamins A, C, K, B5, B6, B2, B3, B1 and E.

Green smoothies for weight loss

Green smoothies have some fantastic characteristics which make them suitable for helping people who are trying to lose weight. The first and most important factor is that green smoothies make you feel full. All of that extra fibre lines your stomach and takes a time to be processed. This means that you are less likely to want to snack between meals and snacks are often very bad for us because they usually contain fats and high sugar content. Then when it comes to the next meal, if you still feel satisfied, you are less likely to want large portions. As a result green smoothies will make you consume less of the junk types of food and less food overall. Green smoothies help to cure cravings for high fat sugary junk foods. These are the same fats and refined sugars that snacks are made from. I have found that not only do I not crave for these types of food but, if I do have them they then make me feel ill. It is as if my body is rejecting them in favour of the natural sugars in the fruit used in the green smoothies.

Green smoothies give the circular muscles of the gut something to work on and this drives the food through your digestive system at a faster rate. This in turn can result in a faster metabolic rate. This is important because a faster rate means that you burn up the food that you have consumed more quickly. People with very fast metabolic rates are the ones that we envy because no matter what they eat they always remain slim. On the opposite side of things those with low metabolic rates are the ones that seem to only have to taste the food to load on the extra weight. Decreasing metabolic rates are the real enemy of traditional dieters. This is when the dieter ends up on a weight loss plateau. Their weight fails to go down no matter what they do. This is a recipe for giving up on a diet and many people do just that. With green smoothies driving you towards a faster metabolic rate you are more likely to stay on your dieting regime and see continuing success.

Green smoothies also contain less fat, and fats are the food group that dieters want to avoid. In addition to this, if fats are eaten in other meals the fibre in the green smoothies will tend to absorb them and prevent them leaving the gut and entering the blood stream.

Although green smoothies contain a lot of carbohydrate it is only the kind that is in the fruit part that is really available to the body. Even this carbohydrate is within cells and has to be processed before entering the blood stream. This means that overall the extra amount of carbohydrate gained is not really a problem. It is slowly released and this means that the body will use it as it comes along.

You can design your green smoothies to reflect the fact that you want to lose weight. However, even if you just throw your smoothies together with the ingredients that are at hand you will find that weight will tend to be lost. If you are making smoothies for weight loss there are certain ideas that you can keep in mind. One of the major things is to use simple recipes. Spring water, coconut water or Rooibos tea is best for the liquid portion but freshly produced fruit juices are equally as good. You should, however, avoid cartons of fruit juice unless they are 100% fruit juice.

Avoid adding a lot of extra fat to your smoothies by not adding such things as nuts and avocado. Some people will also say that coconut is a bad thing, but virgin coconut oils can also increase your metabolism and therefore aid weight loss. You should definitely avoid any hydrogenated coconut products as these don't have the same properties as virgin coconut products. Too much fat in a smoothie can also have unexpected results such as increased gas production and bloating. You should certainly not add dairy products, sugar syrups and artificial sweeteners. The sweetness of the natural fruits should be enough to maintain interest in consuming the green smoothies that you make. The route to smoothie weight loss is to have high carbohydrate and low fat.

Dairy products like creams milk and yoghurts are to be avoided even if they say that they are healthy. These things can contain excess fats and hormones from the animals which produced them. However, if you want to make your smoothie have a creamier consistency then you should add more bananas. Extra sweetness can be attained by using such things as mangoes very ripe bananas and dates. If you are worried about losing calcium due to avoiding dairy you can add such things as dandelion leaves, kale, figs, chia seeds, figs and kiwi. These foods will add extra calcium to your smoothie.

When it comes to fruits you shouldn't use canned or packaged ones because they usually have refined syrup with them. Use fresh or frozen fruits in your smoothie. When times are plentiful you can even freeze fruits for use at a later time. This is one way of having out of season fruits in the winter and saving a little cash.

There are a number of supplements that are produced for adding to green smoothies. These are usually in a dry form and say they will help in weight loss. They are best avoided as they are no longer a pure whole food and are often just driven along by dieting fads. You should concentrate on using fresh products to get the best results.

Although green smoothies can help in weight loss they aren't the whole answer. There still needs to be a lifestyle change to get to where you want to be. One central fact that doesn't change is that true weight loss and management is gained by a combination of a good diet and plenty of exercise. You shouldn't forget the exercise part. However, the green smoothies should increase your energy levels and make you more likely to want to exercise. Don't knock it. This is a good thing.

You can use just about any fruits and vegetables in your smoothies and you will still get results in the weight loss department. However, there are some superstars which you should consider adding to your recipes and these include:

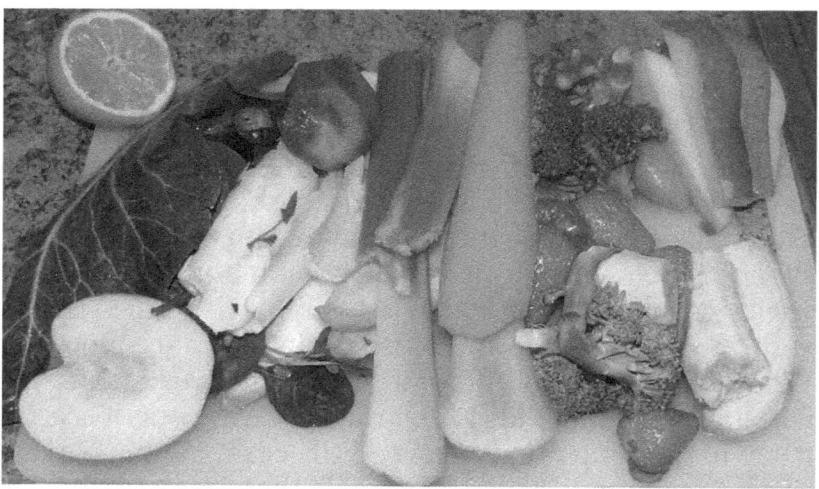

Carrots
Cucumber
Celery
Broccoli

Grapefruit
Pumpkin
Kale
Apples
Blueberries
Pomegranates
Chia seeds
Pears
Raspberries
Strawberries
Bananas

Be careful with grapefruit, if you are on cholesterol reducing drugs such as statins because they can cause a bad reaction which can cause problems with the muscular system. If you are on statins definitely avoid adding grapefruit to any of your smoothies.

To make your weight loss smoothie you should try to use a ratio of 40% fruit to 60% green leafy vegetables and a cup of water. You should see that this ratio has less fruit when compared to the normal smoothie recipe described earlier. This means that there is more roughage from the greens and fewer sugars from the fruit content. All this helps in providing the best conditions for weight loss.

Here are examples of some green smoothies that you can make in order to get your weight loss regime under way. They all have lots of fibre and are low calorie with only small amounts of fat. Simply add the ingredients to your blender and whizz them up for about 30 seconds on a high setting until they are nice and creamy. Don't forget to remove the stone from the peach before putting it into the blender

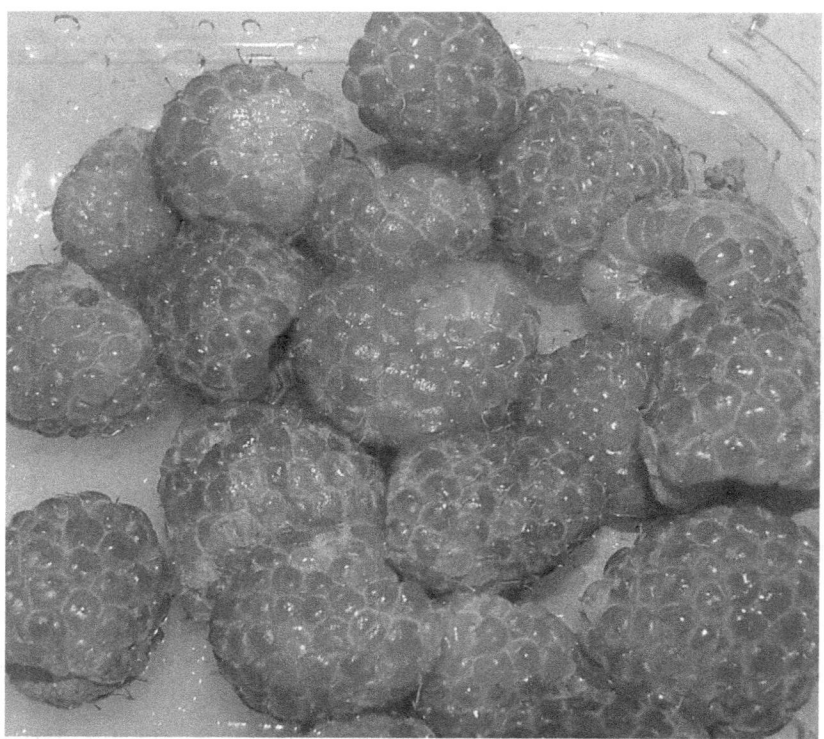

Raspberries

Raspberry and banana green smoothie

1 cup of raspberries
1 medium sized banana
3 cups of fresh baby spinach
2 teaspoons of pre-soaked chia seeds
5 Fluid oz of fresh water

Peach and mango green smoothie

1 one large ripe mango
1 large peach
5 oz fresh baby spinach
5 Fluid oz of fresh water

You can obviously make up your own recipes. These green smoothies are low calorie because the sugars are trapped within cells. If you eat such foods where there is a low density of calories it will be very difficult for you to overeat. The indigestible bulk is the thing that makes you feel full. Green smoothies are a quality food because they have a high density of nutrients but low density of usable calories. These will replace the foods that are really bad for you like fast food, pancakes, waffles and fried breakfast. Instead of eating these you should replace them with a large green smoothie. Carbohydrates aren't bad for you. They are used to provide the energy that your body needs to walk, talk and think. The problem these days is that the food that people usually consume provide far too many of them. The excess ones not used up are then stored as fat. When you try to lose weight you are trying to balance the carbohydrate taken in with the carbohydrate used up by the body doing normal activities. This is where exercise comes in. Extra exercise can use up the carbohydrates and stop them being stored as fat.

However, you should avoid reducing carbohydrates too much. The reason for this is that it causes your body to go into starvation mode. This in turn tells your body to store as much food as it can and also to reduce its metabolic rate. This is the reason that a lot of standard diets fail. You should make sure that you take enough carbohydrate to maintain your body on a day to day basis. In this way you won't end up going into starvation mode. Fortunately green smoothies provide plenty of carbohydrates, to keep your body working, in the fruit portion. You can eat green smoothies when ever you like and you can use them as meal replacements.

Green smoothie detox

Detoxing has become a very popular thing to do these days and there are many commercial products which propose to help you do it. The presumption is that we lead lives which are based on poor health and that every now and then we do something special to put our body systems back on the straight and narrow. I have heard people say that they are going to detox their body because they have had an indulgent week of eating and drinking all of the wrong things. This is all well and good in order to make yourself good for a short amount of time but in reality we should be doing something to keep our body's in peak health all of the time. Green smoothies taken on a regular basis can help to remove and toxins that have built up.

As a result green smoothies could be part of a detox program, if that is what you want, but it is better to change over to a more natural green smoothie diet all of the time. If you are already taking green smoothies on a regular basis they will be doing their job all of the time and removing any toxins.

Toxins or poisonous substances are usually introduced by bad habits such as poor diets or smoking cigarettes. These toxins are usually in the form of chemicals which end up producing free radicals which can damage cells. The magic ingredients for dealing with these free radicals and chemicals are antioxidants. Fruits and vegetables are full of these health giving antioxidants so green smoothies are a great choice if detoxing is what you want to do. You should remember that any detoxing that you do will not be helped if you are still on a poor diet.

When you make your detox smoothies try to select fruits and vegetables with high levels of antioxidants and vitamins. Vitamin C is a good choice and fruits are a natural choice. Use spring water, if you can, as it won't contain chemicals like chlorine. You could even use Rooibos or green tea instead as these both contain lots of antioxidants. Rooibos is probably the better choice because it has the advantage of having no tannins or caffeine in it. It is better to drink Rooibos tea throughout the day and avoid such things as sport drinks, alcohol and sodas. Drinking a lot of this tea or pure water will help to purge your body of toxins as they will be excreted via the kidneys together with the water. The extra water will make you go more often. You should also make sure that you get enough sleep during your detox regime as well. Sleep gives the body a chance to recover and repair itself.

Detoxing using green smoothies will soon have you feeling better as the toxins are removed from your body. As well as this you will feel like you have extra energy and your thinking will become easier and your mind more relaxed.

All green smoothies are good for detox but you can boost their effect by choosing fruits and vegetables that have a particular profile. Adding more fruits will increase the amount of vitamin C which is essential for a good detox. Potassium can be increased by adding more banana, and blueberries are very good as a source of antioxidants. Beta carotene is found in carrots and this is also good to have in a detox smoothie. All you need to do is decide which part of your detox that you are aiming at, and increase the amount of a fruit or vegetable that will supply the right active ingredient.

The recipe below is a popular one that is often used in detox regimes:

1 ½ cups of cold Rooibos or green tea
1 romaine lettuce
3 celery stalks
2 apples
1 banana
1/3 bunch of coriander
1/3 bunch of parsley
Juice of 1/2 a fresh lemon

This particular green smoothie works well at detoxing the liver. This is important because many important metabolic reactions occur in the liver including those used to detoxify poisons. A well functioning liver is reflected in the general health of the body. Coriander helps to deal with heavy metals, if they are in the body. Heavy metals can disrupt important metabolic reactions. The fresh fruit contains many vitamins which often get depleted when the body is run down and having to deal with toxic substances. As well as this it is loaded with antioxidants to deal with free radicals which cause cells to prematurely age. The best way to take your smoothie is as a large glass every morning as part of a general cleansing of the body.

Besides having your usual green smoothies each day you can also go for a detox smoothie at the start of each week. This sets you up ready for the week to come. This could be better for you than just having detox purges. Here is a recipe for one such weekly detox smoothie:

Flesh of 1 lemon
2 pears
2 apples
3 tbsp flax oil
½ tsp of turmeric
¼ tsp of course sea salt
Pinch of cayenne pepper
4 cups cold fresh water

This is a truly remarkable detox recipe which is ideal to have as breakfast on a Monday morning. The lemon and flax oil are really good at detoxifying the liver and at the same time they will help your immune system to work correctly. This is due to the extra Vitamin C and omega 3 fatty acids that they provide. The added turmeric is good for the blood and skin. This smoothie will boost your energy levels, which is just the thing most people need on a Monday morning before they have to trudge off to work. If you like the effects of this smoothie then you could have it more than once a week so that all of your important organ systems are kicked into top gear.

Here are some more detoxifying green smoothies that you can try and integrate into your weekly regime:

Down under detox

2 cups green grapes
3 kiwi fruits
1 medium orange
2 tbsp of Aloe Vera juice
6 leaves romaine lettuce
2 cups cold fresh water

Tropical delight

1 romaine lettuce
1 handful of parsley
 ½ avocado
Juice of 1 lime
2 cups of coconut water
2 tsp of honey

Caribbean garden detox

½ bunch dandelion greens
½ inch fresh ginger root
2 ripe peaches
½ ripe pineapple
Fresh cold water

Green smoothies for energy

Providing extra energy levels for the body has been top of the expectations for green smoothies. In fact the first foods to resemble green smoothies were actually called 'energy soups'. This name came about because of the almost instantaneous boost of energy and mind activity associated with consuming them. This doesn't mean to say that this effect is due to a sugar rush that disturbs the normal blood sugar levels. This would cause problems and is linked to eating foods with too much refined sugar. Rather than being caused by a sugar rush a green smoothie or energy soup provides a whole raft of nutrients in a useful balance. This will of course include some sugars, but also vitamins, minerals amino acids and health giving antioxidants. It is this mixture of nutrients that causes the observed effect on the mind and body.

Sugars are in fact digested and absorbed much more slowly and released gradually. This is due to the amount of fibre in green smoothies. This fibre hangs onto the sugars and the digestive enzymes are forced to work on them more slowly. The vast array of nutrients is made available to the human body by the action of the blender used to produce the smoothie. The blender ruptures the indigestible cell walls of the plant material and releases their soluble contents into the liquid portion of the smoothie. This means that absorption and digestion by enzymes in the gut can take place almost immediately. This is the reason that green smoothies act so fast and make you feel more alive. For some people this feeling drives them on to drink more than the glass of smoothie that they thought they would have. In fact this morning I thought I would have 1 glass of smoothie but ended up drinking 3! This has to be good considering the valuable nutrients in them. It also means that you are unlikely to give up on smoothies like these because they aren't dull. Imagine having to eat the unblended fruit and vegetables. You would soon start to think that the whole process wasn't worth it and stray onto the inevitable meat and dairy products that we are used to. Green smoothies on the other hand will give you steady and reliable energy that will take you through the day so that you can put a whole lot of enthusiasm into the things that you do.

Despite having the same origins, green smoothies are subtly different to energy soups. The main difference relates to the proportions of the ingredients used. Energy soups have large amounts of greens but low levels of fruits. They also have added fats. Green smoothies on the other hand have large amounts of greens and fruits but no added fats. Energy soups can often involve the use of some more obscure foods such as seaweeds. Here is an example of a typical energy soup recipe:

5 cups of baby greens
1 cup of bean sprouts
1 avocado
1 apple
2 tbsp seaweed

These ingredients are then blended in water or apple juice as the liquid content. In this recipe the avocado provides the extra fat content, the apple the sweetness and the seaweed for its high mineral content including Iodine which is essential to the health of the thyroid gland. These days Green smoothie and energy soup recipes tend to overlap but there is still an unwritten rule that large amounts of fruit and fats don't mix easily. As a result as you add more fat orientated vegetables you should reduce the fruit content.

Energy soups could be considered to be more savoury because they have less fruit content and more fat content. You can therefore add other ingredients to emphasise this as well as providing extra health giving properties. For example, you could add a clove of garlic. Garlic by itself is a good natural food, giving boosts to the immune system and also helping to deal with viruses. The above recipe calls for baby greens but if you add more mature leaves you will benefit from more magnesium from the chlorophyll that they contain. More beta carotene and calcium can be gained from using such things as kale, parsley and dandelion greens. For the benefit of children energy soups can be sweetened using banana or raw honey.

The fats in an energy soup can be varied by substituting other fatty natural products such as almond and other nuts. Flax, pumpkin, sesame or sunflower seeds can also be used. You can break up the nuts and seeds by putting them in a coffee grinder before adding to the blender with the rest of the smoothie. Coconut is another good source of fats and you could even add some virgin coconut oil. Virgin coconut oil has a whole raft of extra health giving properties which would enhance your energy soup. It has been shown that adding fats to a diet can help the human body to absorb carotenoid compounds from the gut. Carotenoids are important because they can be converted to vitamin A which is important in a number of metabolic reactions within the body and the health of eyes. Fats also help in the absorption of calcium, iron, zinc and manganese minerals from the gut. It is therefore important to include some plant fats in your energy soups to get the most out of the carotenoid and mineral content.

Green smoothies for kids

There is always a problem in getting children to eat the right things. All young children go through different phases as to what they will and won't eat. My son fortunately loves fruit and will continue to eat it until it is all gone. However, this liking of fruit is balanced by his disliking of vegetables. Just about the only vegetable he will eat is sweet corn. You can guess that we have got through a lot of that over the last few years. However, it is important that children have a variety of greens in the same way that adults need them too. They also need to have a variety of nutrients for their growing bodies. We are encouraged to get our children to eat their vegetables by disguising them and there is no better disguise than a smoothie. Children like fruit juices and my son is always asking for more juice. To children there is no real difference between a smoothie and a juice as they are only really interested with what it tastes like.

Children may question the colour of a green smoothie but hopefully they will soon get over that. It is also good to lead by example. What you are eating they will certainly try. If you do have problems with them associating the green colour with that of the vegetables that they dislike you can start by making mainly fruit smoothies and adding just a small amount of greens. They shouldn't notice this and once you have got them eating them you can slowly increase the amount of greens that you add to the smoothie.

61

Green smoothies are a fantastic way to get your children on the right nutritional path and then to making their own sensible nutritional choices in the future.

By drinking green smoothies your children will get to consume a variety of greens including the difficult broccoli one; take in lots of vitamins, minerals and essential amino acids and eat lots of fresh fruit as well.

As part of encouraging children to make the right choices, you can get them involved in making the smoothies. This is fun and they will love being able to decide what goes into making the smoothie that they are about to drink as well as pushing the button and doing the blending.

You should try to make green smoothies that your children will find appealing and want to drink. Here are some recipes to get you started.

Blueberry and pear delight

3 cups lettuce
2 ripe pears
2 cups blueberries
2 cups water

Tropical summer

Coconut flesh
Coconut water
5 kale leaves
2 nectarines
2 peaches
1 mango

Banana surprise

½ head romaine lettuce
2 ripe bananas
2 oranges
1 mango
2 cups water

Apple punch

5 apples
1 bunch fresh parsley
½ inch fresh ginger root
2 cups of water

Green smoothie hair growth

Hair growth isn't a static thing and as a result there are all kinds of different factors that can influence how well it grows. For a start, hair growth varies according to the seasons with the most growth occurring in the summer. During the year hair goes through cycles of growth and resting. These cycles usually last several weeks. The root is the part of the hair that is responsible for the growth. The roots are part of the skin that makes up the scalp. As a result, keeping the skin and scalp healthy is part of making sure that the hair roots or follicles are kept in good order. They then can produce hair at their best rate. Part of doing this involves supplying them with the nutrients that they need. This is where the nutrient rich green smoothie can come into its own. Here is a recipe for a smoothie that will help to keep your hair follicles in good order.

1 cup water or unsweetened juice
1 cup spinach
1 ripe banana
1 soaked date
1 tsp flax seed

People taking green smoothies on a regular basis have reported that their hair and nails grow faster and that their hair has a better shine to it. It has got to be better to feed your hair for health from the inside rather than pouring chemicals on it to try and do the same job from the outside. I have also experienced more hair growth at the hair line where I had lost hair due to chemical perms and relaxer treatments in the past.

In addition to increasing hair growth some people have found that eating green smoothies can help to deal with greying hair. After drinking a litre of green smoothie a day you could find that the grey colour on a proportion of your hair will gradually start to return to its natural colour. Here is a green smoothie that has had some success in the treatment of grey hair. This one also increases hair growth and shine as well:

1 bunch of dark leafy greens such as kale or spinach
1 cucumber
1 apple
1 lemon
1 inch length of root ginger

You can vary the recipe by using celery instead of cucumber and orange instead of apple. In this way you will get some variety especially if you alternate the dark leafy greens as well.

Green smoothie hangover

If you have been bad and had a night out on the tiles then a green smoothie could be just the thing to get your body and mind back working normally. It can also act as a booster after a hard workout.

½ avocado
½ cucumber
1 ½ cups of chopped kale
2/3 of a sweet apple
1cup fresh water
1 tbsp honey
1 tsp ground cinnamon

Hangovers are typically caused by the build up of toxins in the liver from the alcoholic drinks that you have consumed. They are then made worse by dehydration due to the diuretic action of alcohol in diluting the urine produced. This next smoothie is a good cure for the symptoms of a hangover including headache, upset stomach, tiredness and sensitivity to such things as bright lights and loud sounds.

2 cups of orange juice
1 cup of milk
1 banana
Honey
Ice cubes

The orange juice provides lots of vitamin C and the banana vitamin B which are both good for dealing with a hangover. The milk helps with the upset stomach and the honey both adds sweetness to the drink and boosts blood sugar levels depressed by the hangover. Add sufficient honey to make the smoothie taste nice. You can substitute watermelon for the banana as this also has vitamin B in it.

Green smoothies for acne

The majority of acne treatments involve the application of creams and lotions to the skin surface. While these will often help to remove the visible signs of acne such as blocked pores and inflammation they do nothing to actually treat the reasons for the condition. Acne is usually caused by an imbalance within the body. As a result the only real treatment for the condition will involve treating the internal situation. Green smoothies can help with setting the right conditions within the body for maintaining healthy skin. Only when this is addressed will the acne actually go away. Green smoothies have specific nutrients which can help to clear up acne.

Chlorophyll from the leafy greens in the smoothie helps to purify the blood by removing toxins. This then leads to better metabolism within cells which can result in faster healing and reductions in inflammation of the skin. Vitamin A helps the skin by repairing the connective tissues that make up the bulk of the skin. Sulphur in the smoothie fights infections and reduces inflammation. It also helps to balance the pH of the body. The pH of the skin is important for maintaining a healthy population of helpful bacteria on the its surface. Often these bacteria are the first to go and this allows other bacteria to infect the sebaceous glands and cause the acne. Vitamin K is very good at toning the skin, and in doing so reduces any scarring left by the acne including the red marks on the skin surface. There are also many trace element minerals in green smoothies that are essential for the body but often lacking in modern meat based and cooked diets. These trace elements help many chemical reactions in the body to work efficiently. This in turn has a helpful effect on the general health of the skin. To successfully treat acne you need to make sure that you have your green smoothies on a regular basis. One a day will help with healing and removal of toxins. Having more than one will help to speed up the process further. Carotenoids in green smoothies also help to improve the health of the skin. Antioxidants deal with any free radicals in skin tissue and this helps to maintain the youthful look of skin as well as protecting against skin cancers.

As well as taking green smoothies daily you should also try to remove any acne promoting foods from the rest of your diet. These include such things as refined, sugars and oils as well as dairy products.

The following recipes have proved to be good at dealing with acne problems and clearing skin:

Double dose apple

1 cup apple juice
2 ripe bananas
1 chopped up apple
10 leaves of kale

Mango cure

1 cup water
1 ripe banana
1 mango
10 leaves kale

Papaya tropics

1 cup water
1 ripe banana
1 papaya
1 chopped apple
10 leaves kale

Extra berry

1 cup water
1 ripe banana
1 papaya
1 handful of berries
10 leaves kale

If you can't find kale in your area then you can substitute spinach.

Green smoothie meal replacement

Some people think that green smoothies are the same as ordinary smoothies and are therefore only eaten as a treat or a snack taken between meals. Although they are good tasting and seem to fit the bill we have to really take them a little more seriously. This is because they can be used to meet your nutrient needs throughout the day. This is the case even if you are trying to lose weight on a diet.

A green smoothie may have an energy content of about 500 calories and is therefore the right kind of meal that you need on a diet. For this reason they are ideal meal replacements, especially if you add to this the fact that they are both filling and satisfying. Green smoothies come in a neat package that will provide all of the nutrients that you require. This means that you can stop concentrating on all of the usual dietary concerns such as calorie counting, carbohydrate content, point systems and sizes of servings. This really does free your mind and allows you to enjoy the smoothies that you are drinking.

You can start by replacing breakfast with a green smoothie. The smoothie should be around 400 to 500 calories and if you follow the guidelines stated early this equates to a smoothie that is about 30 ounces in size. When you make up your smoothie make sure that you use lots of nice calorie rich fruits such as bananas, grapes and mangoes. Don't be tempted to pad it out with low calorie fruits such as cucumbers. This is because to get enough calories to make a meal replacement you would have to drink twice as much smoothie for each meal. Whereas a 30 oz smoothie is ok, try to imagine having to drink 2 of them for each meal.

Add to the fruit content about 5 cups of greens. Try to use those that are dark green in colour to maximize the protein content. You can then add a tbsp of seeds such as flax or chia. This then would make a fantastic tasting green smoothie which is ideal as part of a weight loss regime. You can certainly lose weight by just replacing your breakfast; however, if you want to be more serious about dieting then you should try replacing 2 of your meals with green smoothies.

For the liquid in your smoothie use fresh or filtered water or if you would like to, use freshly squeezed juice from fruits. Other dark green leafy vegetables that you can use include dandelion leaves and kale. You should try to include enough of these leafy greens so that the protein content of your smoothie ends up at around 10 grams. These greens will also provide plenty of minerals and vitamins.

Don't use any dairy products such as milk or yoghurts. Don't add a lot of fat containing foods. This will defeat your diet and may also react badly with the fruit causing bloating of the gut and then excess gas. I have had this, and it can get quite embarrassing if you are out working with other people. You have been warned! As a result don't over use such foods as avocado, seeds, coconut and almond butters.

Above all don't make your smoothies too complicated. It is better to concentrate on being simple and adding good honest fibre rich foods. Fibre rich doesn't mean just the green part of your smoothie. You should realize that even fruits such as blueberries, apples and pears contain a good dose of fibre as well.

Here are some examples of suitable meal replacement smoothies that could be used to help lose weight:

Simply Fruit and Kale

2 bananas
2 oranges
3 cups of chopped kale
½ cup of fresh cold water

Plumberry green

2 bananas
4 plums
1 cup blueberries
1 romaine lettuce
½ cup of fresh cold water

Both of these green smoothies have around 500 calories of energy and 10 grams of protein which makes them ideal meal replacements.

Green smoothie for anxiety and depression

There isn't much choice for people who suffer from depressive illnesses in terms of medication. There is no real wonder cure and the medicines that are available tend to treat the symptoms rather than the illness itself. As well as this, all of these medicines have a range of undesirable side effects. You can feel the affects of the chemicals on your body when you use them. The one sure thing is that people wouldn't use them if they didn't have to. This doesn't mean to say that they don't work. I have talked to people who are on these medicines and they say that after using them a while they start to feel better in themselves. Some of the problems of these medicines actually become apparent when you stop using them. In fact a lot of them have proved to be very addictive and as a result it is often very difficult to stop using them when your body is craving them all of the time. Green smoothies on the other hand are completely natural and people often say how calm that they feel after drinking them. This effect seems to come from all of the vitamins and minerals that are loaded into these smoothies. Our bodies know how to use the nutrients and are always trying to be in perfect harmony, and to be as good as they can be. This calmness is a lot different to calmness achieved by using the chemicals in medicines and green smoothies are completely natural without the addictiveness of drugs. In fact green smoothies can help to prevent other cravings for things like caffeine and chocolate. The removal of these things can also lead to a certain calmness as well. You could consider that the calmness of the plants is taken up by the body and is the exact opposite of the caffeine driven fast culture that we are forced to live in. Maybe, it is that we can feel at peace with nature itself through the green smoothies that we are consuming. Either way, green smoothies have got to be worthwhile trying instead of filling ourselves full of chemicals that we are eventually going to get addicted to.

From a scientific point of view deficiencies in essential amino acids in the diet can cause depression and other mental illness. Consuming animal based proteins to get these essential amino acids can lead to deficiencies because animal protein has to be digested first and inefficiencies in the digestive process can mean that some essential amino acids that they contain don't get absorbed. Green smoothies on the other hand contain simple amino acids including the essential ones. These just have to be absorbed by the body rather than being digested. This shortened process is far more efficient. Essential amino acids are used to make neuro transmitters which are important to the working of the nervous system. It is no wonder that a lack of these has been linked to mental illness. It is also thought that nutrient deficiencies can also be responsible for our cravings for caffeine and sugar based snack foods.

Green smoothie oxidation

Some people worry about oxidation processes that occur when you cut up fruit and vegetables during the blending process when you make a green smoothie. The idea behind this is that once you cut a fruit or a vegetable it is exposed to oxygen in the air and that this causes a degeneration of the valuable nutrients within them.

To get an idea of this simply cut an apple into some large pieces and observe what happens as the minutes go by. What you should see is that the cut flesh gradually turns a brown colour. This is caused by the oxidation of phenolic nutrients at the exposed cut surface of the apple. In the same way nutrients like vitamins C will also become oxidised on exposure to the air. This means that as soon as you cut fruits and vegetables the valuable nutrients like vitamins will become destroyed due to reactions with oxygen in the air. This really only happens at the cut surface and certainly doesn't happen with whole fruits that haven't been cut.

The problem is that when you blend a smoothie you are making millions of cut surfaces that expose a greater surface area of the fruit to the air. It would therefore seem that the nutrient content would be dramatically reduced by blending, due to these surfaces suddenly being exposed to the air. However, we have to consider a number of factors here. The first one is that not all of these surfaces are exposed directly to the air as the majority of them are surrounded by the liquid part of the smoothie. This liquid portion will not contain that much oxygen and it certainly won't be replenished very easily once used up. The second factor is that the oxidation process takes time to occur. This means that if you drink your smoothie straight away there will be very little nutrient loss due to oxidation. You stand to lose more nutrients the longer you leave your smoothie standing around.

There are a number of ways that you can go about reducing this oxidation of nutrients. Oxidation is a chemical process and like all chemical reactions it takes place faster as the temperature increases. The opposite is also true in that the speed of reaction decreases the colder that the smoothie becomes. As a result, if you add ice to your smoothie you will reduce the loss of nutrients. If you aren't going to eat your smoothie straight away make sure that you keep it in a refrigerator to slow down oxidation. When you first make your smoothie, make sure that you cut and then blend the fruit and vegetables as quickly as you can. Certainly don't chop them up the night before and then blend them in the morning. One of the ways that cooks use to preserve the vitamin C content of cut salads is to sprinkle lemon juice over them. The acidity of the lemon juice tends to preserve the vitamin C and reduces the oxidation process. As a result adding lemon juice to your smoothie could also help to preserve the vitamin C content. So, it would seem that the best thing to do is to use fresh whole vegetables and fruits; cut them up and blend them quickly and eat the smoothie straight away.

Green smoothie protein

Protein is an important part of our diet. We use protein to make important substances such as enzymes and muscle tissue. Enzymes are the most important of these because they are needed in every cell of our body in order to allow metabolic chemical reactions to take place. These are the chemical reactions of life and without them you can't live. Muscle tissue can be built up by consuming more protein and exercising. This is the reason that weight lifters consume high protein foods and even take protein supplements such as whey powder.

This doesn't mean to say that all protein that we eat is used for these processes. In fact the majority of it ends up in excess and because we can't store protein it is converted to a carbohydrate portion and the waste product urea. It has always been stated that we need to consume food that in total has a protein content of at least 20%; however, these days it is acknowledged that the percentage actually needed is far lower than this in the region of 10%. Proteins are made up of smaller building blocks called amino acids. Proteins are digested to amino acids in our gut before being absorbed by the body. We can make most of the amino acids that we need from any other amino acid in the diet. However, there are a small number of amino acids that we can't make and these need to be in the diet. These are called the essential amino acids. The best way to ensure that you are consuming enough of the essential amino acids is to make sure that you vary the green vegetables that you use in your smoothie recipes.

It doesn't matter if we consume amino acids in the form of complex proteins or simple amino acids. The benefit of taking in simple amino acids is that they are instantly available to the body because no digestion is needed. We therefore waste time and energy when digesting complex proteins. Complex proteins are supplied to us in animal products like meat. However, green leaves supply us with the simple amino acids which don't need ant digestion at all. Once in the body the amino acids are built up into specific proteins that the human body needs at the time. All dark green leafy foods contain high levels of these amino acids and they are generously released during the blending process. You can therefore get enough protein making amino acids from your green smoothies so long as you add leafy greens and vary the ones that you use.

The digestive system breaks down protein included in the diet into the basic building blocks called amino acids. These are then absorbed from the gut and enter the blood stream where they travel to the liver. We can't store amino acids and as a result they have to be dealt with. Those that are needed for protein synthesis are taken up by cells and converted into structural proteins and enzymes for use in important chemical reactions. The rest of the unused amino acids are converted into a carbohydrate portion and the waste product called urea. Urea is then taken to the kidneys where it is excreted together with some water in the form of urine. This sequence means that the extra amino acids from a high protein diet are simply converted into more carbohydrate and waste products that have to be removed from the body. It is therefore better to try and have the right balance of protein in your diet. Eating lots of protein rich foods to excess just ends up creating more carbohydrate that has to be stored as fat and extra stress on the liver and kidneys to deal with the excretory products

There is also research which indicates that consuming a lot of protein in the diet can lead to long term health problems. In particular, research on animals has suggested that high protein diets make them more prone to incidents of cancer in later life. This means that lowering your protein intake to reasonable levels will hopefully allow you to avoid cancer in later life. This evidence has dire consequences for people who have been following high protein diets to try and lose weight. They may in fact be stoking up problems for their body in the future. Leaf protein on the other hand, although in smaller amounts, is easy to digest and is readily taken up from the gut and used throughout the body. Unlike meat protein it doesn't come with all of the associated fat problems

Green smoothie storage

Green smoothies are best consumed straight away to maintain the nutrient content. However, this is not always possible and as a result you can store them in the refrigerator. This will work better if you make the smoothie using iced water and then put it straight in the refrigerator in a sealed container. In this way you can keep your smoothies up to 3 days. Always remember that the nutrients will degenerate over time so the longer you leave then refrigerated the more nutrients that are lost. Adding some lemon juice can also protect some vitamins from degeneration while they are in the refrigerator.

You can also freeze green smoothies ready for later use. Freezing itself doesn't lead to the destruction of nutrients but you should be careful how you defrost your smoothie baring in mind that the warmer it becomes the greater the loss in nutrients. Probably the best way is to transfer the smoothie to a refrigerator and let the process take place slowly.

Green smoothie indigestion

When people first start drinking green smoothies they may experience indigestion and other gastric problems including bloating and the release of gas from the digestive system as flatulence. This is due to the digestive system not being used to the new types of foods and also reactions with the natural bacteria in the gut. This is all part of the natural detoxification of the gut and is quite usual in some people. Over time the gut will get used to the new diet and accommodate it. As a result the indigestion should subside after a while. Problems with excess gas can be caused by the combination of fruits and fats so you should try to reduce the amount of fatty foods like avocados that you add to your smoothies if you experience this. If the indigestion carries on for a long period or you were suffering it before consuming green smoothies you should consult a health professional as it could be an indication of a more serious health condition

Indigestion is caused by the build up of acids in the stomach. There can be numerous causes of indigestion including the foods eaten, acidic drinks like cider, stress and so on. Most indigestion cures use antacids to neutralize the acid content but this can in fact just cause the acid to be produced in greater quantities. Green smoothies are a good cure for indigestion because the digestive enzymes and acid in the stomach tends to be taken up by the fibre in the smoothie. This means that it is not swirling around in the stomach causing problems with the stomach wall and sphincter muscles guarding the stomach entrance and exit.

Green smoothie recipes

Here are some green smoothie recipe ideas. Make sure that you make up the smoothie to the percentages of fruit and green leaves that you want. A typical green smoothie is made up of 60% fruit and 40% green leaves.

Fruity parsley

Mango
Peach
Parsley
Fresh cold water

The parsley gives this smoothie a really fresh taste.

Blueberry ice

Frozen blueberries
Frozen banana
Milk
Yogurt
Spinach
Ground flax seed
Fresh cold water

In this recipe you need to watch how much of the fat based foods that you add.

Orange and spinach

Spinach
Kiwi
Grapes
Freshly squeezed orange juice
Fresh cold water

You can replace the spinach with kale.

Super fruit mix

Kale
Melon
Pineapple
Grapes
Peaches
Strawberries
Blackberries
Blueberries
Raspberries
Fresh cold water

Remember to keep the fruit in the correct proportion to the green kale. Just because a lot of different fruits are listed it doesn't mean that there should be any more than the 60% fruit actually in the finished smoothie. Add water to get the right consistency for your smoothie.

Celery and Mango

1 handful of spinach
1 stalk celery
2 sweet yellow mangos
Fresh cold water

You can use kale instead of spinach.

Herb attack

Spinach
Kale
Parsley
Basil
Peaches
Juice of half a lime
Banana
Fresh cold water

Vary the herbs to get more interesting smoothies.

Berry and weeds

1 bunch red dandelion
1/2 small small watermelon
6 strawberries
1 cup of grapes
Fresh cold water

You can pick your own dandelion in the summer months.

Strawberry kale

1 bunch kale
2 oranges
6 strawberries
1 cup of grapes

Fresh cold water

You can substitute spinach for the kale.

Peach and kale mix

1 bunch green kale
1 pint strawberries
3 small peaches
2 cups water

You can use spinach instead.

Simply spinach and peach

6 peaches
2 handfuls of spinach leaves
2 cups water

A nice simple, but very tasty smoothie.

Zesty kale

4 apples
½ lemon juice
5 leaves of kale
2 cups water

The lemon juice gives a bit of a bite as well as preserving the vitamin C.

Minty kale

4 ripe pears
5 leaves of kale
½ bunch of mint
2 cups water

Try different kinds of mint.

Sweet Romaine

1 cup strawberries
2 bananas
½ bunch romaine lettuce
2 cups water

Romaine lettuce is a good source of minerals and protein.

Weedy mangoes

2 mangos
Lambs quarters weed
Stinging nettles weeds
Purslane weeds
2 cups water

Make the weeds up into a good handful.

Watermelon and berry

One half small seeded watermelon
10 strawberries
1 bunch spinach
1 cup of water

Throw in all the watermelon peel as well as the flesh.

Dandelion and mango

1 bunch dandelion greens
1 orange
1 mango
1/2 banana

You can try other weeds with this recipe.

Tarragon special

Mangos
Strawberries
Kumquats
Mandarin orange
Lambsquarter
Sunflower greens
Tarragon

This is a very delicious smoothie

Cabbage burner

8 oz spinach
8 large Savoy cabbage leaves
1 Whole avocado
3 scotch bonnet peppers
1 red onion
6 cloves garlic
Mint
Parsley

The peppers in this are small but very hot. Be careful with how much you use and vary according to taste. You can also vary the herbs used. A very spicy smoothie for those who aren't feint at heart.

Herbilicious

Basil
Peppermint
Spearmint
Chard
Banana

Try substituting oregano and sage for the herbs in order to get a completely different range of flavours.

Kiwi Combo

Spinach
Kiwi fruit
Banana

A simple but satisfying smoothie with a definite feel good factor.

Spring salad smoothie

½ cup water,
½ cup apple juice
Mixed spring salad
Fresh Pineapple
Red grapes
1 apple
1 Banana
¼ avocado

Use other mixed salad for variety.

Broccoli papaya

2-3 cups broccoli
2 cups papaya
2 oranges
3 dates

You can use any green leaf of your choice instead of broccoli

Minty lettuce

1 handful Cos lettuce leaves
1 handful mint
4 bananas
½ cup water

Try using different kinds of mint. Growing your own mint is really easy as it spreads like a weed.

Winter warmer

1 cup frozen berries
2 cups fresh spinach
¼ inch fresh ginger
Water

The ginger will produce a nice warm glow within you. Use any frozen berries that you have at hand.

Goodbye winter

Fresh orange juice,
Ripe bananas,
Frozen mangoes
Large kale leaves

You can make this a really thick smoothie by adding extra frozen mango.

Apple zest

4-5 kale leaves
4 apples
½ lemons
Water

Add some ice for a really refreshing smoothie.

Baby green delight

2 big bunches of mixed baby greens
2 pears
2 mangoes
1 cup frozen blueberries

Fresh blueberries can be used, if you can get them.

Mock chock mint

2 cups spinach
10 large mint leaves
3 bananas
2 tbsp carob powder
1 cup water

Add more mint leaves for extra flavour.

Celery and spinach

1 handful of spinach
2 stalks of celery
2 bananas
2 pears
1 apple,
1 cup water

You can use kale or broccoli instead of spinach

Green rocket to health

Handful of spinach
2 cups rocket
2-3 mangoes
1 cup water

Rocket is a popular salad item and can easily be obtained from many supermarkets. It has a mild mustard flavour

Lettuce love

½ head romaine lettuce
1 small pineapple
1 large mango
1 inch of fresh ginger

A nice spicy hot green smoothie using healthy fresh ginger root

Dandelion and melon

1 handful wild dandelion
1 small handful mint leaves
3 cups honeydew melon

You can substitute any edible green wild leaves for the dandelion.

Persimmon punch

3-4 stalks celery
2 ripe persimmons
1 banana

Substitute pumpkin for persimmons if you can't get them. However, the pumpkin won't be as sweet as the persimmon

Chard and banana

1 handful chard leaves
6 kale leaves
3 large bananas
1 cup water

You can substitute spinach for the chard in this recipe

Carrot & Kale

Kale
Mixed Greens
2 Carrots
2 Apples
1 Cup Raspberries

The mixed greens could be mixed wild weeds including dandelion

Cilantro cup

Arugula
Sorrel
Cilantro
½ avocado
Banana
Frozen peaches, strawberries & raspberries
Fresh mango
Honey
Water

Cilantro is the same as coriander in European countries

Seeds and fruit

½ banana
½ apple
1 slice pineapple
½ orange
3 dates
2 tbsp flax seeds
1 tbsp dulse
1 lemon slice
1 cup mixed berries
½ cup frozen cranberries
¼ oat bran
1 tbsp sunflower seeds
4 large kale leaves

You can use chard leaves instead of the kale

Curly refresher

Curly kale
½ inch fresh root ginger
½ lemon
Apple juice

Vanilla vortex

Banana
Date
Celery
Kale
Vanilla pod

Vanilla pods are sometimes called vanilla beans

Nutty date

1 tbsp macadamias nuts
2 Dates
1 Small Banana
Spinach Leaves
Water

You can make this one nice and thick and eat it like soup

Radishango

1 large mango
Oranges
Big bunch of radish leaves

Use the whole of the mango including the skin.

Hot & sweet

Pear,
Ginger root
Parsley

The more ginger you put in the hotter it will be.

Mediterranean life

1 bunch of parsley
1 large tomato
½ bunch spring onions
½ lemon
6 green olives
Sea salt to taste!
Water

You can also try adding mint to this recipe. Make it thick as a soup and more water as a smoothie to drink.

Wheatgrass wonder

2 large sprigs of mint
1 handful of wheatgrass
2 apples
2 freshly squeezed limes
1 handful of lambs quarter's, dandelion and lettuce greens mixed
Water
Maple syrup

Double up on the greens mix if you can't get the wheatgrass. Add maple syrup to add sweetness if you feel it is needed.

Lambs quarter and peach

2 cups lambsquarters
2 cups fresh peaches halves
3 cups water

Lambs quarter is a weed so try looking for it. It may even be growing in your garden. Otherwise get a few bunches from a farmer's market.

Blue smoothie

3 cups of greens mix of spinach, romaine lettuce and collards
1 orange
1 cup of Blueberries
6 Cashew Nuts

The blueberries make the smoothie bluer in colour.

Golden smoothie

3 cups of leafy collards
½ cup of pineapple chunks
1 cup of coconut water
6 Almonds

You can use romaine lettuce or spinach instead of the collards

Almond and Pistachio

½ cup almond milk
½ medium banana
½ Cup frozen blueberries
2 tbsp pistachios
1 cup spinach

You can try other nuts in this recipe too.

Lemon Sorrel

½ cup water
6 tbsp ice
1 small banana
½ avocado
3 cups lemon sorrel

If you can't find lemon sorrel then swap it for spinach and add some lemon juice.

Simple Green Carrot

¾ cups carrot juice
¼ cups ice
¼ medium avocado
2 cups spinach

Juice the carrot yourself or buy organic carrot juice. You could always just throw in raw carrots.

Iced grape mix

1 cup grapes
3 bananas
1 orange
5 Cos lettuce leaves
½ cup of water
½ cup ice

You can use other greens instead of the lettuce if you need to.

Mango cream

¼ mango
½ apple
1 banana
1 celery stalk
1 handful spinach leaves
½ cup water
½ cup ice

The banana will make this a nice creamy smoothie

Tropical paradise

½ coconut, water flesh
¼ pineapple
1 mango
3 bananas
¼ cup ice
3 cups spinach

Use a young coconut so that the flesh is nice and soft

Berry mix

1 apple
4 bananas
¼ cup mixed berries
1 cup chopped kale leaves
½ cup ice and
½ cup water

You can use which ever berries that you can get. If you use frozen berries then you can reduce the ice.

Melon Heaven

¼ watermelon
½ of a cantaloupe melon
6 strawberries
9 leaves of Cos lettuce
½ cup water
½ cup ice

You can put in the skin of the melons too.

Peachy

4 bananas
1 cup chopped peaches
1 celery stalk
2 large handfuls of spinach
½ cup water
½ cup ice

Wild and wonderful

1 cup strawberries
3 bananas
1/2 apple
2 cups of wild greens
1/2 cup water
1/2 cup ice

You can use fresh or frozen strawberries in this recipe. For the wild greens consider dandelion, purslane, nettles and if you can't get theses rocket could be used.

Banana celebration

7 ripe bananas
2 celery stalk
2 cups of spinach
1/2 cup water
1/2 cup ice

Use dandelion greens to make a wilder smoothie.

Savoury tomato

1 handful mixed greens
3 Roma tomatoes
1/8 cup cilantro
1/8 cup parsley
1/8 cup basil
1/8 cup dill
1 celery stalk
Squeeze of lime juice
1/2 cup water

Try oregano instead of dill to make a more Italian job.

Herby tomato

2 cups tomatoes
4 Cos lettuce leaves
1 celery stalk
1 handful fresh herbs: basil, cilantro, parsley

Add ice and some Worcester sauce for the perfect hangover cure.

A sniff of garlic

2 Large tomatoes
5 kale leaves
Fresh dill
Lime juice
1 Garlic clove
1 celery stalk
1 slice of red pepper
1 small carrot
1 cup water

A nice spicy smoothie, and you can add as much garlic as you like.

Baby spinach & cream

6 Bananas
1 Apple
4 cups baby spinach
1 cup water
½ cup ice

The bananas will blend to a lovely creamy consistency.

Up the Blues

1 cup chopped mango
4 bananas
2 cups spinach
½ cup blueberries
½ cup sunflower sprouts
1 cup water
1/2 cup ice

The more blueberries the bluer it gets.

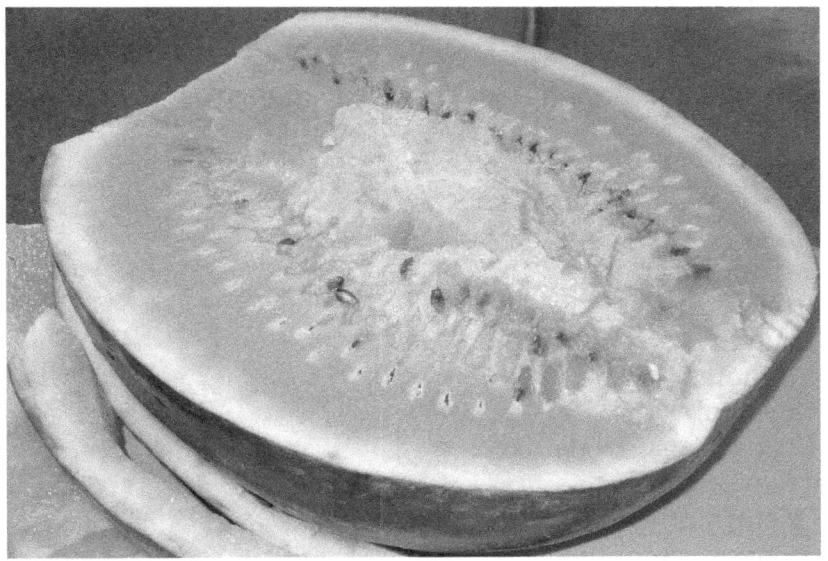

Watermelon patch

12 cups watermelon
6 cups chopped Cos lettuce leaves
Water
½ cup ice

The water melon has a lot of liquid content so be careful with the amount of water added. Add banana for a thicker and creamier result.

Spicy tomato

2 cups chopped tomatoes
½ cup of tomato juice
¼ cup apple juice
½ cup carrots
¼ cup chopped celery
Hot pepper sauce to taste
2 cups ice

Use a Caribbean hot pepper sauce such as Tabasco or Encona.

Seeds and vegetables

2 tbsp balsamic vinegar
4 tbsp salsa
1 cup raw broccoli
1 tomato
½ carrot
1 cup chopped kale
2 cloves garlic
½ cup sunflower seeds
½ cup sesame seeds
2 slices onion

Use sunflower seeds where the seed coat has been removed. You can substitute fresh lemon juice for the balsamic vinegar.

Broccoli Boost

1 carrot
4 broccoli florets
2 handfuls of spinach
1 apple
2 oranges
Orange Juice

Peel the oranges or throw the whole thing in. It is up to you.

Strawberry cantaloupe

½ cantaloupe
1 cup strawberries
2 cups spinach
¼ cup fresh water

You can cut the rind from the cantaloupe or throw the lot in.

Berry cantaloupe

½ cantaloupes
1 cup organic raspberries
2 cups fresh organic baby spinach
¼ cup fresh water

You can use blueberries or blackberries instead of the raspberries or use a mixture

Grape cantaloupe

½ cantaloupe
1 cup red grapes
2 cups baby spinach

You can use other fresh greens instead of the spinach. There shouldn't be any need to add water.

Apple and cantaloupe

½ cantaloupe
1 apple
2 cups baby spinach
¼ cup fresh water

Why not use pear instead of the apple.

Nectarine and cantaloupe

½ cantaloupe
1 nectarine
2 cups baby spinach
¼ cup fresh water

You can use peach instead of nectarine. In either case don't forget to remove the stone from the fruit.

Watermelon detox

1 carrot
2 cups chopped watermelon
1 banana
3 cups chopped kale
1 orange
Fresh cold water

In this smoothie kale and watermelon come together to make a fantastic detoxifying combination.

Green turnip

1 large handful of turnip greens
1 cucumber
1 mango
1 banana
3 cups of fresh cold water

There are lots of vitamins and folic acid in turnip greens so make sure you add enough of them.

Kid's choice

1 banana
1 cup grapes
6 oz vanilla yogurt
1/2 apple
1 1/2 cups fresh spinach leaves

You can use plain yoghurt instead of the vanilla one and adding strawberries can make it more interesting for children

Bok choy and cinnamon

2 apples
1 teaspoon of ground cinnamon
2 tangerines
1/4 avocado
2 heads of baby bok choy
6 oz fresh cold water

Apple and cinnamon is a classic flavour which is made nice and creamy with the added avocado.

Bok choy and parsley

2 bananas
1 cup of chopped pineapple
1 cup fresh parsley
2 heads of baby bok choy
6 oz coconut milk

The parsley makes a really good combination with the pineapple which makes this green smoothie very tasty.

Red cabbage and Blueberry

2 cups chopped red cabbage
1 cup blueberries
2 medium bananas
2 teaspoons soaked chia seeds
6 oz fresh cold water

This smoothie makes an interesting change in colour to the usual green one. Dark red and different with all of the usual cabbage properties.

Red cabbage and grapefruit

1 grapefruit
1 cup chopped red cabbage
1 banana
6 oz fresh cold water

Peel and deseed the grapefruit for the best results with this purple smoothie.

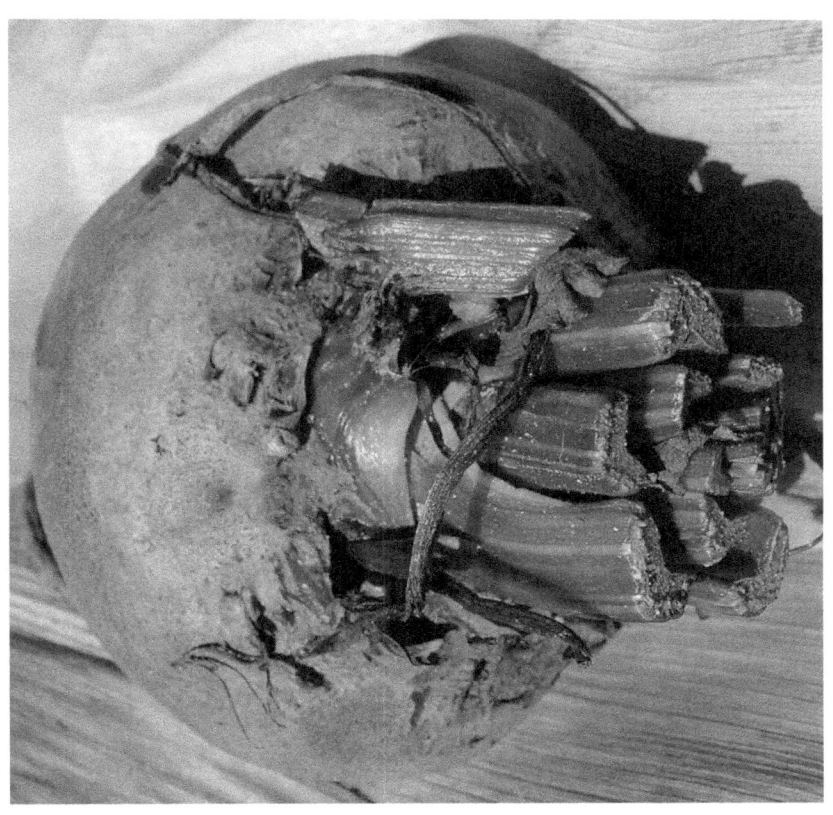

Beetroot and fruit

1 beetroot
2 cups spinach
1 date
1 chopped apple

A nice red and green smoothie. Peel the beetroot before blending

Red-Red

Red cabbage
Cos lettuce
Carrot
Strawberries
Ice
Water

There are lots of red and orange colours in this smoothie.

Spicy beetroot

Pineapple
Carrot
Celery
Beetroot
Ginger

Add more ginger for a more warming smoothie

Cucumber and ginger

Cucumber
Kale
Apple
Mint
Lemon
Ginger

The more cucumber you add the fewer calories that the smoothie will have.

Orange and fennel

Orange
Carrot
Kale
Ginger
Fennel leaves

Add fennel seeds for extra aniseed flavour

Beetroot and parsley

Beetroot
Parsley
Kale
Carrot
Apple

Beetroot and parsley make a nice herb and root combination

Chocolate milk

Kale
Almond milk
Banana
Raw cocoa

Make sure that you use raw cocoa for the best results.

Spinach and minty cucumber

Spinach
Cucumber
Apple
Mint
Lemon

Add the lemon to make this as zesty as you like.

Chocolate cream

Raw cacao,
Frozen banana
Spinach
Almond milk

The banana and almond milk make this a very creamy smoothie.

Banana berry

Berries
Banana
Spinach
Soy milk
Honey

Use a variety of berries or one single kind. You could choose from raspberries, blueberries, strawberries etc.

Carrot and cinnamon

Apple
Carrot
Ginger
Celery
Cinnamon
Water
Ice

Cinnamon has many health giving properties all on its own so it is well worth adding to your smoothies.

Wild water melon

Coriander,
Mint
Watermelon
Wild greens

Coriander is a unique flavour that will really set off your selection of wild greens such as dandelion, purslane and lambsquarters.

Cucumber and lime

Baby spinach
Orange
Lime
Ginger
Cucumber

Give cucumber a real zest with this fruity number.

Kiwi and cucumber

Baby spinach
Kiwi
Cucumber
Mint

Kiwi and cucumber add a very light juicy flesh to this smoothie.

Cucumber and celery

Spinach
Cucumber
Mint
Kiwi
Celery

The celery and mint add an interesting dimension to this cucumber based smoothie.

Banana Brazil

Banana,
Spinach
Kale
Celery
Brazil nuts
Water

Interesting flavour is added with the use of the Brazil nuts.

Conclusion

Choosing to drink green smoothies is both a health and a lifestyle choice. In doing this you are making your life a green and happy one. Green smoothies can help your body and life in all kinds of ways from dieting to dealing with anxiety and mental disorders. Green smoothies deliver the power of nature straight to your body without added chemicals or chemical processes such as preservation, cooking or artificial flavour enhancing. All of the extra nutrients that your body gets to use can help you fight all kinds of diseases by keeping your immune system in tip top condition. This means that your body is better equipped to fight any disease organisms as soon as you come into contact with them. Green smoothies can make you feel fitter with greater levels of energy for both your body and your mind.

The first thing you notice is that green smoothies taste a lot better than they initially look. The fact that they taste so good makes it easier to carry on drinking them. Most diets involve you eating things that aren't as interesting as green smoothies. In order to carry on long term with green smoothies it is important to try making lots of different ones to maintain your interest. This will involve a lot of experimentation on your part but the end results will be well worth it. You can also react to local seasons so that you don't have to buy things that are out of season and more expensive. The Green smoothie diet doesn't have to be an expensive life style change.

The idea of meal replacements can help you control your diet. You can choose to replace one meal or 2 meals of the day with green smoothies. How far you go is entirely up to you. When you replace a meal you should make sure that you drink enough of the green smoothie to get through to the next meal. This will take a bit of experimentation but if you drink only a small sized smoothie you will find that you will feel hungry and this is when you are most at risk of snacking on foods that aren't good for you.

It does take a while to get used to drinking green smoothies because your digestive system has to learn how to deal with them. This may lead to an initial period of bloating and flatulation. After a while your body learns how to digest them and your system will return to normal. In the initial stages you should pick when it is most convenient to have your smoothies. I remember going to work on the first few days with my stomach churning away as it worked on the new diet. You just have to remember that this should be a temporary thing.

Once you are well into your green smoothies you will definitely start to see all of the benefits whether that is losing weight or just getting the buzz of out of your body and mind having the nutrients that they deserve. This feeling of well being is what we all deserve so don't forget to pass on your new found zest for life, and how to get it, to your family and friends.

About the Author

Ellen Vincent has seen at first hand the differences that whole natural foods can make compared to the pre-packaged, processed and sanitized food that we eat in the west. In her native Ghana food comes straight from the field and is prepared in traditional ways.

Since living in the West she has sought to avoid the new foods that were presented to her and has embraced more natural diets. Green smoothies provide an excellent way of bringing these natural ways back into your life. She has found that there are great benefits to be gained from eating the raw foods included in green smoothies. After experiencing better health of body and mind from green smoothies she was determined to show the rest of the world how they too could gain a better and healthier lifestyle.

Ellen is also interested in the natural care of hair and skin. She produces her own skin and hair care products from natural ingredients. These products have proved to be very successful and she is determined to produce a further book to show how these products can be combined with the benefits of green smoothies to produce a complete system where skin and hair are kept in perfect condition by conditioning them from both the inside and outside of the body.

When thinking about our health and well being, you have to consider the fact that we really don't understand how all these modern chemical additives and treatments are affecting the human body. In the future people may look back in horror at what we have managed to do to ourselves, in much the same way that we view the use of poisons such as arsenic and red lead in cosmetics in the past. The best thing to do is to stick to the healthy options that come from the plants around us. Use the shea butter, coconut oils and other natural products because they have served us well for thousand of years and have never let us down. In all things, nature and not necessarily science and technology seems to know what is best for us.